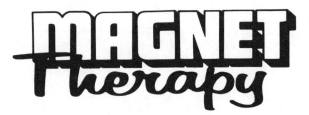

MAGNET Therapy

How magnetic applications can help your aches and pains.

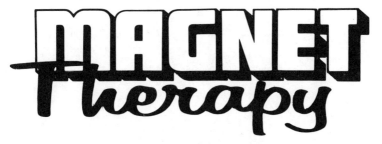

How to Use the Healing Power
of Magnetism to:

soothe pain

steady the nerves

increase metabolic activity

treat a variety of ailments

by

E. Holzapfel, P. Crépon, C. Philippe

Translated from the French by Transcript

THORSONS PUBLISHING GROUP
Wellingborough * New York

First published as *La Magnéto-thérapie* by Editions Retz,
Paris
First published in the United Kingdom 1986

British Library Cataloguing in Publication Data

Holzapfel, E.
    Magnet therapy: how to use the healing
    power of magnetism.
    1.   Magnetism — Therapeutic use
    I.   Title   II. Crepon, P.   III. Philippe, C.
    IV. La magneto-therapie. *English*
    615.8′ 45   RZ422

    ISBN 0-7225-1185-X

Printed and bound in Great Britain

CONTENTS

1.

MAGNETISM

A Little History

According to legend the properties of the magnet have been known since the day they were accidentally discovered by Magnes, a Greek shepherd.

He was taking his sheep to pasture when, on passing a large rock, he found his iron-mounted staff being pulled towards it by an unknown force. He had to exert all his strength in order to tear it away. This rock was named the Magnet Stone. It is said that, being very amazed by the force and wishing to make use of it, he inserted pieces of the stone inside the soles of his sandals ... and that this enabled him to cover long distances at one stretch without feeling tired.

This makes a nice little story, but we may be quite sure that the magnet was used for curative purposes well before the times of Ancient Greece. In fact, it would seem that most of the old cultures, especially those of the Chinese, Indians, Egyptians, Arabs and Hebrews knew the use of the natural magnet. It was especially employed to make amulets. There is no doubt that these were thought to safeguard good health and to repel bad influences from those who wore them.

Aristotle (third century BC) was the first person in history to talk about the therapeutic properties of the natural magnet, called by him the 'white magnet'.

In the first century AD Pliny spoke of the use of the magnet for diseases of the eyes. Galen, in the third century, extolled the virtues of the magnet as a cure for constipation. And Marcel, a French philosopher and physician of the fourth century, recommended wearing a magnet on the neck to relieve headaches.

Alexander of Tralles in the sixth century employed a magnet in the treatment of painful joints, and Avicenna in the eleventh century used it against melancholy. About the same time, Albertus Magnus was claiming that the magnet exercises a powerful and salutory effect on the system.

Apparently, the magnet was used almost continuously right into the sixteenth century, when Paracelsus could still cite its usage. He seems to have been the first to mention polarity. Even though his description is rather vague, he does say that he applied one or the other end of the magnet according to the effect sought.

Kircher, the celebrated German Jesuit scholar, published many writings on the magnet and in particular his *Magnetismus medicinalium*, in which he informs us of the continuous utilization of magnets since high antiquity. He describes the methods employed and the results obtained.

Subsequently, numerous physicians and scientists have persevered in using the magnet and in publishing their findings on it. Father Hell, a famous astronomer, manufactured magnets in a variety of shapes and sizes to fit human limbs.

For a while during the eighteenth century the abbé Le Noble, canon of Verneuil-sur-Seine, made a careful study of the applications of the magnet in the treatment of diseases. In 1777 he sent the Société Royale de Médecine a dissertation on his work. The Society appointed two experts, Audry and Thouret, to 'verify the efficacy of the magnet in the treatment of diseases'. The two commissioners performed their task with the most scrupulous attention. The detailed report they published contains not only an account of the experiments on maladies but also an important compilation of the previous researches. The findings of the report are so favourable to this 'new therapeutic method' that the only reservation expressed by Audry and Thouret concerns the risk of making it a panacea. They conclude that, 'the magnet seems one day destined to play as big, or at least as essential, a part in medicine as it now plays in physics'.

Interestingly enough, a few years later, the Société Royale de Médecine, which had sponsored the work of Audry and Thouret, condemned the 'animal magnetism' championed by Mesmer.

After six years, the same commissioners drew up for the Société Royale de Médecine a second report containing sixty-one fresh observations of different cures due to the application of magnets. In 1843 Eydam published a thesis on 'the application to the human body of a magnetic field for therapeutic purposes. Then, in 1869, Maggiorani announced the positive results obtained by applying magnetic fields to the human body in the treatment of patients suffering from hysteria, ataxy and diabetes.

Charcot and Renard, in 1878, utilized the action of magnetic fields in the treatment of hysteria.

Paul Spiegler in his *Bibliography of the Biological Effects of Magnetic Fields* (1962), cites numerous other works dating from 1900 to the present day, but he does not seem to have been aware of the interesting publications on the subject issued between 1900 and 1930 or thereabouts by the French naturopaths Hector-Henri and Gaston Durville, or of the writings of Dr Leprince.

Magnets and Magnetic Fields

The rock that attracted the iron tip of Magnes's staff was composed of ferromagnetic minerals. Such rocks are often volcanic: the lava flowing during an eruption cools slowly and is then imprinted by the earth's magnetic field. When the lava is cold it contains a certain quantity of magnetic energy.

The sites where the biggest deposits of ferromagnetic minerals are found are in the arctic regions, in the north of Sweden, Finland, Greenland and Siberia.

The mysterious force possessed by natural magnets appears to have fascinated mankind ever since its discovery. Without doubt, it was with the idea of appropriating this force that man has made amulets and jewels containing fragments of natural magnet. As we shall see, this idea based on intuition and observation was not so unfounded as might be thought. Nowadays ferromagnetic minerals or natural magnets are virtually no longer used as such; artificial magnets are preferred mainly because for a given volume they are more powerful.

It is easy to make a magnet. Take a piece of iron or steel and place it inside a coil of insulated electric wire, or just wind an insulated wire several times round a nail. Pass the current from an ordinary battery through the wire for ten seconds, and the iron is then magnetized.

The Earth's Magnetic Field

The earth behaves like an enormous spherical magnet with a north pole and a south pole. The energy of a magnetic field circulates between the two. It is now known that this field is not constant but has varied during the earth's history.

There are some scientists, notably professors Kawai and Rikitake in Japan, who claim that the earth's magnetic field is continually decreasing in intensity. Kawai 'estimates that the force of terrestrial magnetism has diminished by 50 per cent in the course of the last five centuries and by 5 per cent in the last 100 years'. However, their assertions are contested by other scientific researchers, who say that although the earth's field may have weakened it could regain strength during the coming centuries.

Dr Prime of the American Insitute of Geology, resuming the work commenced in 1906 by Brunhes, a French physician, has examined the lava on the sides of a certain number of volcanoes. Brunhes discovered that the lines of force inside magnetic rocks had changed direction relative to the north-south axis. According to the depth at which these lines are situated in the rock, he could establish the periods when these changes of direction were produced. He found that the earth's magnetic poles had changed places several times in the past.

Using carbon dating, Prime was able to determine at what epochs these reversals of polarity had taken place. Recent investigations relying on carbon-14 dating of marine or terrestrial animal fossils have supplied additional evidence: significant changes in existing species and the appearance of new species have coincided with changes in the intensity of the earth's field and with inversions of the poles.

Anyway, if other causes still unknown were not operating at exactly the same times as the said changes — and it is highly improbable that they were — we are fairly safe in assuming that the earth's magnetic field directly influences life and evolution.

Nakagawa, to whom we shall return later, goes so far as to think that the present weakness of the earth's magnetic field is creating a serious magnetic deficiency which is harmful to all living species and is responsible for countless illnesses.

Polarity

There is a well-known experiment in which a magnetized needle is placed on a cork disc freely floating in a bowl of water. One end of the needle turns to point approximately in the direction of geographic north and the other in the direction of geographic south. This property of polarity is, of course, what makes compasses useful. A magnet is *always* polarized and therefore always has a north pole and a south pole. One pole cannot exist alone but invariably implies the presence of the opposite pole. *

It is easy to confirm that in a length of magnetized iron or steel wire, one end forms the north pole and the other forms the south. No matter how many times we cut the wire up, this phenomenon will always recur.

To identify the poles correctly is important, because, as we shall see, each has a specific effect and because many of the magnets sold commercially are wrongly marked. The simplest method is to obtain a bar magnet or a cylindrical magnet. The bar or cylinder is suspended by its middle from a wire or thread in such a way that it is able to turn freely. After its oscillations have come to a stop, one end of the magnet will be pointing towards geographic north and the other will be pointing towards the south.

* This is certainly true of the poles in ordinary magnetic materials, but some scientists suspect that there may be such things as independent magnetic monopoles and are trying to detect them.   (Translator's note.)

The end that turns towards geographic north is the south pole of the magnet, and the end that turns geographic south is the north pole of the magnet. *

It is necessary to paint or otherwise mark an 'N' on the north pole of the magnet and an 'S' on the south pole.

The orientation of the bar magnet obeys the law that like poles repel and unlike poles attract one another. And so the north pole of our globe attracts the south pole of the magnet and vice versa.

Once we have at our disposal a magnet the polarity of which we have verified and permanently marked, it is easy for us to find the polarity of any other magnet by the simple application of the above law that like poles repel and unlike poles attract.

Modern Magnets

Up to World War II most of the magnets made artificially were of soft iron, like the horseshoe magnets sold in shops. But, in relation to its mass, soft iron is unable to store more than a relatively modest amount of magnetic energy. Consequently, in order to obtain the required strength, we are obliged to employ very large and heavy magnets, which is hardly practicable.

The Durville brothers used for curative purposes cloth jackets studded with magnets and weighing several pounds. The bracelets were equally heavy and cumbersome. But now we have magnets which not only are more powerful but are smaller and lighter into the bargain.

The composition of these modern magnets is complex, and it includes metals such as nickel, cobalt, tungsten and even for the most recent ones rare earths such as Samarium, Cerium, Yttrium, etc. Our most powerful magnets have an intensity of magnetization which can be as much as fifteen times greater than that of the classical ones. What is more, the new magnets have greater retentivity, meaning they become demagnetized more

* **N.B.**   The naming of the poles in this book is the opposite of the traditional British system, which calls the 'north-seeking pole' the 'north pole' for short.   (Translator's note.)

slowly than did the old magnets, for which reason we call them 'permanent'.

Since these second and third generation magnets (the latter being the 'rare earth' magnets) are both less bulky and much more powerful, great strides have been made in magnet therapy. They have made possible the advent of Taiki therapy, of which we shall speak later in the book.

How the Electrons are Aligned

When a piece of iron is placed in a coil carrying an electric current, the iron becomes a magnet, as we have already seen.

So what has happened? The electric current has simply rearranged the atoms in the piece of iron. With the atoms now in alignment, the electrons are orbiting in the same direction. The magnet's field strength depends on the induction of the atomic nuclei and thus, on the number of atoms that can be polarized in this way. End on, the magnet presents us with a vortex of electrons, rotating clockwise or anticlockwise according to the end being viewed. The rotation is anticlockwise at the magnet's north pole and clockwise at its south pole (remember that here the north pole is the British south pole and vice versa). In other words, the rotation at the north pole is 'sinistrogyric' or leftward turning, and the rotation at the south pole is 'dextrogyric' or rightward turning.

The ordering of the electrons during magnetization musters and deploys energy which was previously potential, when the arrangement of the electrons was haphazard.

Now there is a mistaken idea, still taught in most of the text books, that the flux of energy leaves the south pole of the magnet and flows without more ado to the north pole.

It is to the research of Albert Roy Davis and Walter C. Rawls that we are indebted for exact knowledge of the way in which the magnetic circuit behaves.

First of all, we should understand that the classical experiments on the form and arrangement of the magnetic flux described in our physics or electricity books are often based on false premises. In fact, to determine the pattern of a magnet's lines of force, the method generally adopted is to sprinkle iron filings on a sheet of glass. Then, when a magnet is placed underneath the glass, it is seen that the filings form definite tracings. The next step is to assume that the so-called 'lines of force' seen in the tracings give a description of the energy flow. But this is not so at all. The experiment is incorrect in its conception, because it does not allow for the fact that each particle of iron placed in the field of the magnet becomes a tiny magnet in turn and therefore attracts and repels the neighbouring particles. Thus the picture presented by the iron filings is definitely not representative of the way in which the real flux moves in space, but is the composition of this flux and of the individual flux of each particle of iron.

Thanks to the many precise measurements made at their research laboratory in Green Cove, Florida, Davis and Rawls have managed to give a more adequate description of the actual circulation of the magnetic flux.

It is interesting to observe that their laboratory work has been confirmed by work carried out by the National Aeronautics and Space Administration of the USA (NASA) when making precise measurements of the earth's magnetic field at various degrees of latitude and longitude.

Without overcomplicating matters, here are the main points for the reader to bear in mind. The old, erroneous theory said that the magnetic flux issues from the south pole and pursues a direct route to the north pole. This was supposed to be just as true of the earth's magnetic field as it was of an ordinary magnet. It is illustrated in the drawings opposite.

In reality each magnet, including the earth, has a middle zone where the magnetic field is zero.

For a spheroid like the earth, the zero zone is the geographic equator — as has been demonstrated by field work performed by America's NASA. In this neutral part, the sense of rotation of the electrons reverses. In other words, the vortex which is revolving to the right as it leaves the south pole rejoins the earth's surface in the equatorial regions where its sense of rotation reverses through 180°. Then, revolving to the left, it proceeds to

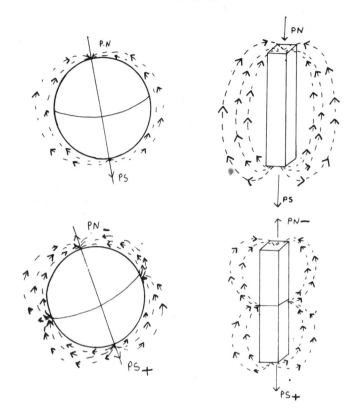

the north pole and re-enters. The same is true of any other magnet. (See diagrams.)

So the idea that magnetism flows in a single direction is wrong and not in keeping with recent scientific discoveries, according to which, as we have seen, the magnetism of a magnet flows in two directions.

Energy Loss

Part of the magnetic energy leaving the poles does not return to the magnet (or to the earth, as the case may be). The magnetic waves emitted in this part, which are (one should remember) rotating either clockwise or anitclockwise according to their pole of origin, travel in nearly straight lines. They move out a great distance from their pole and fail to return to the magnet. On this showing, the earth's magnetic field is bound to weaken with time. In the same way every other magnet will gradually lose energy. Since we are tolerably certain that this is what does happen, we conclude that the earth's magnetic field was once stronger than it is today.

Space technology has shown that leaving the earth's magnetic field to enter a weaker magnetic environment can affect astronauts quite seriously. In other words, a significant diminution in the terrestrial magnetism that bathes all living beings will badly disturb the processes of life.

Man-made magnets are subject to demagnetization too, but our modern ones lose strength very slowly. One way of retarding the loss still more is to close the circuit by joining its two poles with a conducting wire. The magnetic energy then circulates with hardly any loss through the ring that has been formed.

On the other hand, every time a magnet is employed to pick up a piece of metal, for example, some of its energy leaks away into the metal to which it is applied. In general, any physical contact made by a magnet results in a loss of energy by transfer to the body with which it is in contact. This is even so when a magnet is placed on any part of the skin for healing purposes.

2.

THERAPEUTIC EFFECTS OF MAGNETS

Before examining the work relating to the strictly therapeutic uses of magnetism, it may be helpful to make a rapid review of work on other applications carried out in certain countries. Indeed, the field of study is so large that most of the major nations have cultivated it.

Often the interest has been military. Joint studies made by French and Russian teams have shown, for instance, that fish find their way be means of a magnetic guidance system which could perhaps suggest ways of improving the guidance of missiles. Other experiments made in England, Germany and the USA have led to the same conclusions where birds are concerned. One experiment involved suppressing their sense of orientation by fixing a magnet near the head of migratory birds.

The United States are especially interested in those aspects of magnetism connected with astronautics and, in particular, in the problems created for man in space by weak magnetic fields.

Countries vary considerably in the degree of attention devoted to the effect of a magnetic field on living organisms — known generally as 'biomagnetism' or, in the USSR, as 'magnetobiology'.

The Russians seem to be making considerable headway here. Since 1948, Red Army doctors have used magnets to reduce the pain in limbs after amputation. Research into this aspect is being carried out mainly at the Medical Insititute of Rostov and at Leningrad Military Academy.*

In Canada, research is being led by several universities in

* *Cf.* Davis and Rawls, *The Magnetic Effect.*

conjunction with the Ministry of Agriculture with a view to improving germination by exposing grain to magnetic fields. A 10 per cent better harvest is anticipated.

It seems that Japan is the country where most attention is being paid to the therapeutic uses of the magnet. Some experiments have been conducted in hospitals. The Japanese Ministry of Health has given its approval to several types of bracelets or necklets containing magnets and now on sale to the public through chemists' shops.

The Research of Nakagawa in 1976

Nakagawa's research involved the use of a magnet 5 mm in diameter and 2.5 mm thick, which was almost the size and shape of a lentil.

The magnet is attached to the skin by a piece of round sticking plaster some 1 cm in diameter. The magnetic field measured by contact with the magnet is 590 Gauss. Although Nakagawa does not mention the fact in his study, it is important to mention that this type of magnet (the use of which is very widespread in Japan) is always supplied with the south pole (British north pole) of the magnet stuck to the plaster so that the north pole (British south pole) of the magnet will be in contact with the skin. In employing the magnet, one simply attaches it to the painful area of the skin, or to any area which is stiff or tense.

A questionnaire was sent to 11,648 users, who stated their sex, age, the symptoms for which the magnet was used, the results and how long it took to achieve them.

In general, the magnets were used for the following painful conditions:

Stiffness of the neck and shoulders	45.20 per cent
Lumbago	19.00 per cent
Neuralgia	13.90 per cent
Painful muscles	12.30 per cent
Rheumatism	1.30 per cent
Other	6.30 per cent
No reply	2.00 per cent

Women made up 57 per cent of the total and men 43 per cent. The age group most represented was from 40 to 49 years. Out of the entire population used in this study (11, 648 cases), more than 90 per cent said that the procedure was effective for treating the indicated symptoms. The comments of this 90 per cent can be summarized in three categories (though Nakagawa himself does not categorize them):

— 'Very efficacious'

— 'Efficacious'

— 'Fairly efficacious'

Finally, less than 10 per cent regarded the product as 'ineffective' or 'not very effective'.

Usually, the effects make their appearance on the second and third day of use. More than 90 per cent of the effects classified as 'efficacious' appeared before the end of the fourth day. No negative effect such as aggravation of the symptoms was reported.

Other Japanese studies have been analysed by Dr Pierrick de Kerdaniel in *Les cahiers de biothérapie* of March 1980.

There were four studies, all made in 1976. One was by Professors Akio Yamada and Shuwichi Hirose of the Faculty of Medicine of the University of Tokyo. The second was by Professor Yamamoto of the University Juntendo of Tokyo. The third was by Kyoshi Kurushima of Kohnodai National Hospital, and the last was by Nakagawa, who carried out the study already cited. The article tested was a necklet in which the magnets delivered 1,300 Gauss on contact. In some studies a double blind test with a placebo was employed (certain subjects received unmagnetized necklets, and the doctors and subjects did not know which necklets were the magnetic ones until after the results had been collected). The main symptoms for which the necklets were worn were pains in the back of the neck, and in the shoulders, back, arms, hands and legs. Approximately four hundred subjects took part in the four studies.

According to the comments of Dr Pierrick de Kerdaniel

on these careful studies, three important points stand out:

- The effectiveness on the given symptoms of the magnetic field supplied by the necklets is quite evident, and falls within a range of 60 to 80 per cent.

- The harmlessness of the product was proved: there were no side-effects and physical examinations did not reveal any biological changes that might be attributable to wearing the necklet.

- The time limit for the action is between the seventh and the fourteenth days. (We note that this is longer than that given in the first study by Nakagawa mentioned above.)

Finally, Dr de Kerdaniel analyses a study by Dr Yoshio Ooy on a belt containing magnets delivering about 1,500 Gauss on contact and designed to relieve lumbar pain. The test involved eighty subjects, fifty of whom received a belt with magnets of the stated strength, and thirty of whom received a belt with less powerful magnets (200 Gauss). The following results were obtained.

With the full-strength magnets, sixty-two subjects showed a very marked improvement, a marked improvement or a minor improvement (we do not know the exact break-down into these three categories).

With the weak magnets or placebos, no subject showed very marked improvement but 23 per cent showed marked improvement or minor improvement (once again we do not know the exact break-down).

It is worth quoting de Kerdaniel's conclusions at full length:

> The only view we can take of these figures and of the scientific care with which this study was undertaken, is that we are in the presence of one of the most interesting therapeutic procedures it is possible to study; a procedure in which acupuncture plays a part. Essentially, the magnets are arranged on the plastic body-sheet in such a way that when it is properly belted on they lie over the two branches of the Bladder Meridian and over the Tou-mo Meridian.

We would comment on this set of Japanese studies as follows:

1. The greatest effect is seen in Nakagawa's first study, in which magnetic pellets were used.
    Next in value was the lumbar belt, then the necklets.

2. None of the studies mentions polarity.However, as already stated, the pellets (study No. 1 by Nakagawa and the magnetic belts for lumbar pain) are always supplied with the north pole (British south pole) in contact with the skin.

Even though the pellets were about half as powerful as the magnets in the belts or necklets, the results obtained with them were quicker as well as better. In the case of the necklets the north and south poles acted simultaneously because the magnets were placed horizontally on the skin.

We shall come back to these findings later and to the implications it is possible to see in them. But for the moment, let us content ourselves with noting that many of the subjects, especially those taking part in the experiments of Yamada and Hirose, remarked that in addition to affording relief from the troubles for which they were employed, the magnets imparted a sense of well-being and produced an improvement in their general health.

The Effects of the Two Poles on Living Beings

It is now time to return to the very important work of Davis and Rawls. We have already mentioned their revised concept of the magnetic field, but the reader may find it worthwhile going over its essential features once more.

The magnetic energy supplied by each of the poles differs both in potential and in value. The vortex or rotary flux of the electrons is clockwise on leaving the south pole (British north pole) and anticlockwise on leaving the north pole (British south pole).

The north pole (British south pole) is *negative.*
The south pole (British north pole) is *positive.*

In the centre of a magnet there is a neutral zone where the sign and the sense of rotation of the electron flow is inverted. Some of the energy emitted by each pole streams far out in a straight line and does not return to the magnet. However, another part of the energy travels from the south pole (British north pole) to the equator (or to the centre of a bar magnet) and then from the equator to the north pole (British south pole).

So, do the north and south polarities produce identical effects on living matter, or not? In their work, Davis and Rawls relate how in 1936 they tested this aspect by accident. Thousands of other experiments followed, the most important of which were reproduced in other laboratories.

Some of Davis's assistants who were going fishing had collected earthworms *(phylum annelida)* in three cardboard boxes and had put them in the laboratory. One of the boxes was unintentionally placed close to the south pole (British N.P.) of a large horseshoe magnet. The live worms had been left with a sufficient quantitiy of good damp soil in each of the boxes. Holes had been pierced in the boxes for ventilation, but the lids were on tight to prevent the intended bait from escaping. Because some unexpected work cropped up, the fishing expedition had to be cancelled and the boxes remained where they were in the laboratory for some thirty hours.

Two days later, when the would-be anglers came in to pick up their bait, they were greatly surprised to find that the worms in the box next to the south pole (British N.P.) of the magnet had eaten one side of their cardboard prison. Various experiments followed with earthworms placed in boxes made of stronger cardboard to prevent escape. In this series of tests, the boxes were placed in contact with magnets for periods of twelve days.

Those in contact with the north pole were marked N, while those in contact with the south pole were marked S; finally, a third group marked C were used as a control.

The findings were as follows. The worms in the boxes marked S (which had been in contact with the south poles

(British north poles) of the magnets) were full of activity and were busily engaged in eating the inside of their cardboard box. They were approximately a third as large, both in length and diameter, as the worms in the control group. What is more, the soil contained a number of freshly hatched worms.

In the boxes marked N (which had been in contact with the north poles [British south poles] of the magnets) a great number of the worms were dead, and the survivors were thin and displayed little activity. Those in the boxes marked C (the control group) did not appear to have undergone any appreciable change. The authors gradually refined their tests, using different intensities with different exposure times and different forms of magnet – in particular bar magnets, which have a better separation of the north and south energies than that found in the horseshoe magnet, since the poles are further apart.

A biological examination of the treated worms revealed a considerable increase in protein amino acids in group S, no change in group C, and a considerable reduction in group N. Thus the energy of the south pole (British N.P.) encouraged the production of protein amino acids, and the size, activity and physical strength of the animals.

A large number of experiments were then carried out on seeds. The results were very varied according to the exposure times, the strength of the magnetic field and the species. The other variables, such as temperature, degree of humidity and soil quality were carefully controlled. The seeds responded like the worms. The plants that were bigger than those in the control belonged to group S, and those that were smaller to group N. The plants in group S, whether they were green vegetables, fruit, tubers such as potatoes or root crops like beet, all showed big effects in a large number of tests in which they were exposed to the positive energy. Generally speaking, the quantity of oxygen liberated was more than the carbon dioxide absorbed. The size and weight of the plants was greater than that of those in the control group, and the period of growth was usually shortened. There was an improvement in the general metabolism of the plants. The beet yielded more sugar and the peanuts more oil. In group N the effects were exactly opposite: smaller size and weight in comparison with the control group, slower growth and weaker metabolism.

Davis and Rawls conclude that we are dealing here with two types of energy. One inhibits life, growth and development, while the other improves activity, metabolism and growth.

Their conclusions are worth comparing with the observations mentioned earlier, according to which important mutations in living species and/or the appearance of new species coincide with big changes in the terrestrial magnetic field.

Finally, a great number of tests were performed on animals, hens' eggs, mice, snakes and birds. Those interested in the details of the test are referred to the works and report of Davis and Rawls; it would take too long to describe everything here. Let us just say that these tests lead to the same conclusions as do the tests on worms or seeds, as far as activity and an increase in metabolism, size, weight etc. are concerned; and that the effects of the two poles are the inverse of one another in the same way.

However, what is more interesting still is the distinctive behaviour of subjects exposed to the positive energy. They display more intelligence and adaptability than do the members of the control groups and frequently assume the role of leaders. In the tests on mice and rats the males in the S groups showed an increase in sexual activity and, in some cases, this excessive sexual activity was such that the males killed the females by their roughness.

The Magnetic Mother

One last test deserves mention.

Newly hatched chicks were put in coops. The coops were comfortable and contained water, food, and a floor-covering of soft soil. The eggs from which these chicks had been hatched were previously exposed to north or south magnetic fields.

The coops were labelled N, S and C (according to whether their inmates had been exposed to north or south energy (British S or N energy) or belonged to the control groups). Inside each of the coops was a horseshoe magnet 15cm long with a 5cm gap between the poles; there was also a dummy (placebo) or imitation magnet of the same size as the real magnet and painted in exactly the same colours.

The chicks in group S, while still not dry from the egg, turned towards the magnet and installed themselves one by one between its poles. After remaining there for some two minutes each removed itself from the magnet and went to the other end of the coop. Another chick then placed itself between the poles of the magnet for the same length of time and withdrew. This behaviour was repeated until all the chicks had taken their turn. At no time did any chick approach the false magnet of wood!

The three sets of chicks — S, N, C — behaved in the same way with slight variations.

The chicks in group N, whose eggs had been exposed to north (British south) magnetic energy during incubation, remained between the poles somewhat longer than did those exposed to energy from the opposite pole.

The chicks in group C waited until they were quite dry before going to the magnet. Theirs was the longest stay between its poles and lasted between $2\frac{1}{2}$ minutes and $3\frac{1}{2}$ minutes.

The bogus magnet did not attract a single chick from any of the groups.

This experiment is interesting in several ways. It shows that the chicks have an innate, untaught perception of the magnetic field as a source of comfort and strength. The experiment has been called that of 'the magnetic mother' because the chicks automatically go to the magnet as they would go to the mother hen for her protection, support and warmth. It is interesting too that the birds in the three groups all behaved in the same manner — even those in group C, which had never been in contact with magnetic energy during incubation.*

---

* Except, of course, for the earth's magnetism. (Translator's note.)

Tests on Tumours and Cancers

In concluding this section, it is necessary to say a word on the long series of tests performed by Davis and Rawls on cancerous tumours. For a period of eighteen years they experimented with the effect of magnetic fields on the development of tumours and cancers.

Here, in brief, are their main findings on rats, rabbits, mice and other animals; for the most part, they used the technique of transplanting cancerous cells into healthy animals.

Whether the growth was in its early stages or was more advanced, it appears that when the magnetic energy of the north pole (British S.P.) was applied to the affected area the pathological condition improved and the development slowed down or stopped. According to the authors, these improvements occurred in more than 90 per cent of cases depending on the stage of the disease, and on the age and physical condition of the animal.

Counter-experiments were performed by exposing the cancerous sites to south (British north) magnetic energy. The invariable result was an aggravation of the pathological condition and a more rapid development of the tumours.

In addition, healthy animal tissue was exposed to north (British south) magnetic energy before the transplantation of the cancerous cells. The groups of animals treated in this way displayed a remarkable increase in resistance to the success of the cancerous graft and to its development.

Hypothesis Concerning the Way Magnet Therapy Works

Several ideas plainly emerge from a reading of the above:

— the application of a static magnetic field has an incontestable curative and beneficial action;
— the percentages of good results obtained in the different studies cited are high;
— the harmlessness of the treatment seems to be well established;

— in addition to the therapeutic results under immediate investigation, numerous patients in several of the studies talk of a feeling of general improvement.

But how does magnet therapy work?

Nakagawa and the 'Deficiency Syndrome'

Dr Nakagawa, whom we have already mentioned, is the author of many works on magnet therapy. He has analysed the results of numerous experiments for over twenty years and puts forward a theory he calls 'the magnetic field deficiency syndrome and its treatment'.

The following are the main points of his theory. The earth develops a stationary magnetic field known as the terrestrial magnetic field. According to several recent scientific reports, to which we have referred earlier, the strength of the terrestrial magnetic field may well have decayed by 50 per cent during the last five centuries, and the weakening is continuing at the rate of 5 per cent per century; hence the terrestrial field should be zero in 2000 years.

Nakagawa warns that since man has been living in this magnetic field from time immemorial, the change is likely to entail organic disorder. He adds that modern life in a world of iron, steel and concrete deprives us of yet more of the already insufficient terrestrial magnetism. Cars, trains, and ships in particular screen us from its beneficial action.

This is why he speaks of a veritable 'magnetic field deficiency' responsible for numerous human disorders. The principal symptoms are stiffness of the neck, shoulders and back, lumbago without radiographic evidence, chest pains without any precise cause, persistent headaches, drowsiness, giddiness, insomnia, constipation, lassitude, etc. Because the application of magnets relieves or removes these troubles in a great many cases, Nakagawa thinks there must be such a thing as a 'magnetic field deficiency syndrome' and that the deficiency may be made good by the application of a magnetic field. This hypothesis is intriguing, and there is probably more than a grain of truth in it.

The reader may remember the disorders suffered by the astronauts during their time spent in space in a magnetic field much weaker than that on earth. The occurrence of these disorders tends to bear out Nakagawa's contention, but we cannot be certain that the weaker magnetic field really was the cause of space sickness, let alone that it was the sole cause.

In any event, some people would maintain that the disorders described above are the well-known 'diseases of civilization'. Also, as we have seen, amulets, jewels and pendants made of magnets have been used since high antiquity ... when the earth's magnetic field was much stronger than it is today.

Then again, if Nakagawa's hypothesis is correct, the pathological effect of the weakness of the terrestrial magnetic field ought to create disorders in animals as well as in man. Nothing suggests that this is so.

Barnothy

Barnothy in *Biological effects of magnetic fields* (New York 1964) speaks of a thermomagnetic effect and of an electromotive force created by electromagnetic induction in a liquid. This force probably exerts its strongest action on the blood.

Other researchers, such as P. Fabre and A. Collin, cited in Nakagawa's study, have put forward explanations of the same type involving a magneto-hydrodynamic effect on the circulation.

Davis and Rawls

The leading ideas in the explanations proposed by Davis and Rawls, while not contradicting the theses of Nakagawa and Barnothy, seem more convincing.

They regard the living cell as a 'system in electrical equilibrium'. Any change in the cell's electrical equilibrium will tend to deform or damage it. It is now possible to measure the volts on the external surface of a blood cell, and the first sign of trouble is an increase in the negative voltage. The charge on the blood cell in bioelectric ions is the result of the charges represented by sodium and potassium ions. This charge and its level depends on the selectivity of the cell membranes. Any change in the bioelectric charge on the membranes modifies the charge on the cell itself, so affecting its balance and health.

Davis and Rawls noted after prolonged investigation that in every case, whether animal or human, where 'internal repair' was going on, there was an increase in the negative bioelectric potential on the external surface of the affected region.

Upon recovery of health, the negative potential drops and returns to normal. Should it fall below normal, this is always a sign that the part affected has not succeeded in regaining its equilibrium. In cancerous cells, for example, the negative potential is much less than normal. The same applies whenever there is some physical injury — such as a broken limb, say. The body's own healing processes are invariably accompanied by a temporary rise in the negative potential.

Specific Effects on Pain

One of the fields of application where magnetotherapy (and, above all, Taiki therapy) comes into its own is sedation, that is to say, the suppression or alleviation of pain.

Davis and Rawls propose the following explanation. The tissue cells and blood cells carry an external negative charge due to sodium and an internal positive charge due to potassium. On the other hand, the nerve fibres carry an external positive sodium charge and an internal negative potassium charge. This, of course, is exactly the reverse of the charges in the other tissues and in the blood.

When the nerve terminals are affected by an abnormal situation such as pressure, infection, burns, etc., they inform the brain of the danger. If negative magnetic energy (that coming from the north pole — British S.P.) is applied, there is a reduction in the external positive potential on the outer envelope of the nerve fibre, and this has a sedative action produced by the diminution in the sensitivity potential of the positive ions. Therefore, in general, the application of the negative magnetic potential reduces nerve sensitivity (thus acting directly on the pain) at the same time as it assists self-healing; which, as we have seen, always involves an increase in the negative bioelectric potential.

Dr Bhattacharia and Dr Sierra in their *Power in the Magnet to Heal* have added to the explanations of Davis and Rawls. After making numerous measurements, they have shown that in different parts of the body the skin has an electric charge that is positive, negative or zero. For example, they state that the highest positive voltage on the front surface of the body is found in the region of the heart and has a value of approximately 70 microvolts.

The voltages and skin sites as described by the authors can vary a great deal from person to person. They also vary in the case of disease; but with the help of magnets the correct potential can be restored wherever it has been disturbed.

In closing these few remarks on the possible mode of action of a magnetic field on pain and/or disease, we would stress that in the majority of cases it is the negative energy that is required and that this exerts a double action:

(a) the sedation of pain;
(b) intensification of the curative activity, which is always accompanied by a temporary increase in the negative potential.

Nevertheless, utilization of the positive energy from the south pole (British N.P.) of a magnet could be justified in some instances.

The Different Types of Magnets Used in Treatments

A variety of magnets are used for therapeutic purposes. All we can do here is to mention the main types and to indicate those which are commercially available. *

The most important factors as far as therapeutic use is concerned are the following:

---

*   The author adds: 'in France'.   (Translator's note.)

— the strength (measured in Gauss)*;
— the ratio of strength to mass;
— the resistance to demagnetization (the degree of retentivity).

As we saw earlier, soft iron magnets are scarcely ever used nowadays. Because their strength-to-mass ratio is small, they have to be too big and cumbersome to be practical. What is more, they demagnetize relatively quickly.

The improved composition of modern magnets has given them much greater strength and also has much improved their strength-to-mass ratio and their retentivity.

These factors are more or less prominent depending on the exact composition and mode of manufacture of the magnets. It should be noted that the manufacturing cost of permanent magnets that are very powerful for a small volume and have great retentivity is still high.

Shape is also an important aspect. According to whether the poles are well separated or close together, they can be used singly or as a bipolar unit.

The Necklets

Magnetic necklets have been tested for a long time in Japan and are now being marketed in Europe. They consist of eight to twelve rare-earth magnets arranged longitudinally round the neck, and individually supplying a bipolar flux of 1,300 Gauss per magnet.

Each magnet is a cylinder about 12.7mm long and 3mm in diameter.

Taiki Items

These items are characterized by being polar and self-contained.

* Strictly speaking, the 'magnetic flux density'. (Translator's note.)

In fact, in the usual model, which is 5mm in diameter and 2.5mm thick, the magnet is mounted on a round adhesive plaster. Thus it can be placed accurately on any spot that is sensitive, sore or unwell.

Magnets of this type were employed in Nakagawa's study No. 1 described on p.18. As we have seen, such magnets achieved the highest percentage of success as well as the greatest rapidity of action.

It seems reasonable to ascribe the excellence of these results to two main facts:

— the polar action is superior to the bipolar action;
— the localized action is quicker and better than the non-localized action.

These two factors are what differentiate Taiki therapy from magnetotherapy. Otherwise, the magnets supplied by Taiki owe their effectiveness to a moderate strength on contact of approximatley 600 Gauss, whereas the belts and necklets (especially the latter) deploy at any given time a higher unit force from a number of larger magnets.

Finally, Davis and Rawls state in their writings that they manufacture therapeutic magnets in their Florida laboratory. At the same time, they disclose few details and do not mention the sizes and characteristics of their magnets. They do, however, mention 'advanced' research on 'VHG' (Very High Gauss) magnets, i.e. very powerful magnets of 20,000 to 100, 000 Gauss!

They think that the application of magnets of this strength would be likely to cure various ills and to arrest the development of any form of cancer completely. Obviously, we have to treat such assertions with great caution for the moment.

We are informed by the firm of Taiki that they intend marketing curative magnets of 1200 to 1500 Gauss, with the same characteristics of polarity and of self-sufficiency as their 600 Gauss magnets. They are available from:

Acumedic Centre
101 Camden High Street
London NW1 7JN

Medi-Swiss Ltd
21 Crowsley Road
Shiplake
Henley-on-Thames
Oxon

A range of magnetic products is available from:
Healthways Products Ltd
28 Richmond Hill
Bournemouth BH2 6EJ
Telephone: (0202) 28986

It is now time to take a look at the relationship between magnetotherapy and Chinese medicine with its various stimulotherapies.

3.

STIMULOTHERAPIES

A wide variety of therapies exist for treating disordered organisms. Thus, certain chemical or natural substances may be prescribed to act on the internal organs direct: a method widespread in the West and representing one of the foundation stones of our medical practice. Another method consists of working on the external envelope of the organism, that is to say on the skin and superficial muscles.

Therapy of the second type is little used in the West except for massage to re-educate the muscles. Lesions and weaknesses of the organism are thought often to have an internal origin, which suggests the necessity of treating them at this level. In fact, it might as well be admitted that occidental medicine tends to regard the superficial layers of the body as no more than a very thin envelope for the whole ultra-complex of tissues, organs and circuits that they protect, and to imagine that their role is limited.

However, another great medical tradition, which has been developed in the Far East, has to do with therapeutic treatments that act on the epidermis. We shall return to these stimulotherapies later, simply making mention here of acupuncture, moxa (stimulation by heat), and oriental massage. *

The Chinese have elaborated a very complex system, which explains how action on the skin and superficial

---

* It should be made clear, that Chinese medicine does not neglect internal medication, and has a highly sophisticated tradition of herbalism.

muscles can affect the internal organs through energy circuits. Since some knowledge of the system is indispensable for understanding how Taiki therapy works, it will form the subject of the following chapter. But first we must take a closer look at the envelope of the human body and at the various ways in which it may be stimulated.

Man is linked to the universe, with which indeed he is completely interdependent. This prime truth, which was known to all the great traditions of antiquity, has been partly forgotten during some centuries of burgeoning Western medicine. And even though the most recent scientific discoveries such as chronobiology have once more brought it to light,it has not yet been restored to its rightful place in our thinking.

It would be ridiculous to see man in isolation from his environment. The perpetually changing universe is always acting on him, by cosmic radiation, sun-spots, the rhythms of the sun and moon, the changing seasons, weather patterns and many other external influences in his daily life. As part and parcel of this universe, man is a complex organism with his own special physical, mental and energy characteristics. In other words, he is a microcosm living in and interacting with the macrocosm or universe. The body's envelope is the boundary between the two and, thanks to this privileged position, does much to preserve the harmony between them.

Imagine a funnel with one opening representing man and the other opening the universe, and suppose for a moment that the narrow neck connecting them is the outer covering of the human body. For the human machine to function properly it must fall into line with the laws of the universe, and this desirable state of affairs can be achieved by deliberate action on the skin and superficial muscles or, in other words, on this narrow link between microcosm and macrocosm. It is essential to keep well in mind this strategic role of the body's envelope because, all too often, Westerners assume that acupuncture and other stimulotherapies operate only through laws linking the cutaneous points with internal organs. They do operate in this way, of course, but we need a wider outlook. For instance, there are electromagnetic fields involved, and a human being will be in good health if his body's electromagnetic field is stable in itself and is in balance with the electromagnetic waves of the entire cosmos. The surface of the body plays a decisive part in maintaining this overall equilibrium.

The Specificity of Certain Cutaneous Points

The skin with its underlying parts is rather more, however, than the boundary between the internal system and the external world. It contains a number of points having definite properties. These points were discovered several thousand years ago by the Chinese, who grouped them along lines called meridians. They gave them pride of place in re-establishing the proper functioning of the internal organs and in harmonizing them with the cosmos. When acupuncture became known in the West, researchers attempted to discover a physical reality in these points which, until then had been conceived in terms of energy alone. Their idea was to find an objective basis for Chinese medicine. Some workers looked for electrical properties, others for a distinctive morphological structure.

The electrical properties of the Chinese acupuncture points
The first investigation into the electrical properties of the Chinese points was carried out by Dr Niboyet of Marseilles, who made it the subject of his doctoral thesis presented in 1963. His work has been followed up and his results have been confirmed and recognized.

It would be tedious to describe here the whole of Dr Niboyet's experimental procedures, so we shall content ourselves with reviewing his essential findings while referring the interested reader to the original publications. * But what do we mean when we talk of the electrical resistance of the human body? 'It was the German physician, G. S. Ohm who gave the first clear account of electrical resistance and his name to its unit of

* The most recent, with bibliography, is in the *Nouveau Traité d'Acupuncture* (Editions Maisonneuve, 1979).

measurement. Electrical resistance is the electrical characteristic of a body that adjusts the intensity and the power of a current to one another. However, Ohm's law defining this resistance applies to inanimate matter and does not seem valid in the case of the human body.

Thus, in metals, for example, the measure of electrical resistance is practically a constant. But in the human body the measures of electrical resistance display numerous variations. The localization of the measurement on the body is one element entering into these variations, but there are several other significant parameters too. In order to show that certain precise points on the skin have some special electrical characteristic, it is necessary to make a sufficient reduction in the influence of the other parameters.

Various experimental procedures were used for this purpose. For instance, the pressure of the electrode as it was applied to the points had to be controlled so that pressure variations would not falsify the results. Also the presence of phenomena of spontaneous electrolysis — arising from the secretions of the skin or from some other electrolyte — required countering (measurements were taken under a current of alcohol). Finally, the areas of skin tested were carefully examined for any microscopic injuries that might interfere with the experiments. All these precautions did enough to reduce the number of disturbing causes to ensure that the differences recorded in the measurements were due soley to differences in placement on the skin. The results are totally convincing and highlight the fact that the cutaneous points and lines of energy (meridians) linking them, as described by the Chinese, have a physical existence measurable in terms of electrical resistance.

Here are the conclusions of Dr Niboyet as expressed in his latest work: the *Nouveau Traité d'Acupuncture* (New Treatise of Acupuncture) (1979, p. 239–240):

After a considerable number of measurements had been taken, the researches showed:

—   The existence of points of least resistance (between 20 per cent minimum and 50 per cent plus) in certain areas of the body's natural covering. The origin of these 'pits of minimum resistance' does not seem to be assignable to classical factors.

— These points of least resistance are arranged symmetrically on the right and left sides of the body (with the exception of the points situated on the median lines).

— If two points are measured between two punctiform electrodes, the resistance is always weaker when the two points are 'in line' (i.e. when they belong to the same meridian). So there are paths of least resistance. They are symmetrically disposed on each side of the body.

A comparative table setting the traditional Chinese teachings side by side with our own findings, will allow some conclusions to be drawn.

Chinese tradition	Experimental findings
1. In precisely determined zones in the body's cutaneous covering, there are individualized invisible points, differing in their action from the integument surrouhding them.	1. In the acupuncture zones described by the Chinese, there is always a point of least electrical resistance. This difference in resistance from the surrounding integuments is a significant one, yet does not seem explicable by the classical factors.
2. The majority of these points (that is to say all the points, except those belonging to the single meridians on the median lines of the body) are symmetrical on the right and left sides of the body.	2. These points (except for those situated on the median line of the body) are always found to within a millimetre at symmetrical places on the right and left sides of the body.

3. Most acupuncture points are not isolated entities, but on the contrary are joined by more or less straight lines, called 'meridians'.

3. The resistance is always less between two points in a given meridian than between these and any other point, whether the latter is an acupuncture point in another meridian or is just taken at random. In other words, between two points in the same meridian runs a path of least electrical resistance.

4. The meridians have two branches situated on the two symmetrical sides of the body (except for the single central meridians).

4. The paths of least resistance are found on the symmetrical right and left sides of the body.

5. In certain circumstances and under certain conditions, these points have physiological properties when stimulated by a slight traumatism.

5. The verification of this statement is partly attempted in part three.

The analogies encountered between Chinese tradition and experimental findings in the course of our research are too numerous and too constant to be put down to simple coincidence. We are therefore led to conclude that the points of least resistance situated symmetrically on the right and left sides of the body, inexplicable as they are in terms of classical anatomy or physiology, can be assimilated to the Chinese acupuncture points. There are also paths of least resistance to electricity on the skin following the same routes as those of the meridians.

The morphological structure of the acupuncture points
Investigations aimed at finding a special morphological structure of the skin at the site of the acupuncture

points, are much less conclusive than those relating to the points' electrical properties.* Actually, these studies are too recent for proper verification and their results are not accepted by all. We cite them merely by way of information.

The Korean, Kim-Bong-Han, for instance, believes he has succeeded in detecting a specific structure for the Chinese points, but the structures he describes have been rejected by the French writers. On the other hand, some Austrian researchers interested in the same problem have reached negative conclusions concerning the existence of a specific structure.

More recently, Professor Sénelar has carried out research along the same lines. Experiments he has performed on rabbits have led this author to think that there is a significant neuro-vascular structure at points of least electrical resistance. However, it is much too early to reach conclusions, and further work will have to be done to determine if the cutaneous points traditionally described by the Chinese possess any special morphological features.

Various Methods of Stimulation

Having underlined the fundamental importance of including the envelope of the human body in a general view of man and the universe, and having discovered the existence of cutaneous points with special properties, we now come to examine the various methods of stimulating these points.

To begin with, there are three main traditional methods which Chinese medicine has been using for thousands of years: acupuncture, the moxas, and massage. To these we must add other secondary measures, all of them traditional: the cupping glass and the instrument known as the 'plum tree flower', for example.

In addition, modern techniques have introduced other

*   See Sénelar: 'Les caractéristiques morphologiques du point chinois' (The morphological characteristics of the Chinese acupuncture point) in *Nouveau Traité d'Acupuncture* (Maisonneuve, 1979).

means of stimulating the skin. These seem rather promising, in fact. Among them must be mentioned techniques utilizing electrical energy (electropuncture), sound waves (sonopuncture), laser beams and the electromagnetic field (magnetotherapy and Taiki therapy).

Acupuncture
This is the best known form of stimulotherapy and its name has become a generic term for all the Chinese methods of cutaneous stimulation. Acupuncture consists of the insertion of needles at precise points. The act of inserting the needle in the skin while observing a certain number of laws for finding the correct point of insertion is called the puncture.

The needles come in various shapes and sizes according to the point where insertion is to be made and to the desired action. Traditionally there were nine types of needle but others have been used since. The material from which the needles are made does not seem to be critical, because in prehistoric times the Chinese employed needles of stone, bone or bamboo. Nevertheless, the needles are always made of metal nowadays. Usually they are of stainless steel, but sometimes are made of silver or gold. Apparently the results obtained are different with one or other of the latter materials.

Acupuncture is certainly one of the most effective of the stimulotherapies and for this reason it is reserved for specialists. It is out of the question for a person who has not been trained in the theory and practice of Chinese medicine to perform acupuncture. Each point has to be perfectly located with a very fine needle, and the latter needs to be manipulated in different ways according to whether a tonifying or dispersant effect is required.

Also, it must be emphasized that in certain cases, where young children or the elderly are concerned, or in certain diseases, acupuncture may prove difficult to apply. But then other stimulotherapies can take its place.

The moxas
The moxa technique consists of utilizing heat to stimulate the cutaneous points. This procedure is at least as ancient

as acupuncture and is very widely employed in the Far East. To make moxas, little cones of mugwort (artemisia) powder are placed on the acupuncture points; these cones burn slowly, without flame, something like a stick of incense, and emit a growing heat. To avoid burns, another method is adopted in which a large 'cigar' of mugwort is brought close to the point being treated without touching the skin.

Stimulation with moxas is as efficacious as acupuncture but has its own special virtues. For example, it is recommended when rheumatic diseases or certain symptoms such as fatigue are present, and for diseases where acupuncture would not be tolerated.

Acupuncture can be combined with moxa by using heated needles. For this purpose, practitioners employ special needles having a cavity at one end filled with mugwort. More simply, they can use needles with a ball-shaped head designed to be heated with a cigarette lighter.

Moxas, and certainly the heated needles, are usually left in the hands of specialists, just as is done with acupuncture. However, the mugwort 'cigars' which are easier to use and have a gentler effect, can be self-administered by patients who have been shown exactly which points to treat.

Massage

In the Far East the development of massage has taken a different course from the one taken in the West. It has drawn on Chinese medical theory and, in simplified form, its use is widespread among the population.

Several techniques can be distinguished. Some, like Do-in, are of Chinese origin; others, like Shiatsu, belong to the Japanese tradition. They all utilize special points in the body which are stimulated by pressure. However, these techniques are not limited to a simple routine of applying pressure to various points. There are several different pressure techniques and considerable experience is required in selecting the right ones. For instance, a tonifying pressure is quite unlike a dispersing pressure. Then again, such massage includes various types of movement and friction for improving the general circulation of energy without involving the stimulation of any particular point. It will easily be understood that, in the circumstances, a genuine massage which is really effective has to be based on long practice and special talent.

On a lower level, the massages can be used simply as a way of stimulating the points by hand. Massages of this type are used in the Far East and also in the West , where for some years acupunture has become very fashionable. Stimulation of pressure points with the fingers is undoubtedly effective; nevertheless we ought not to be too casual. On the one hand, it is still necessary to distinguish between the dispersing action and the tonifying action and, on the other hand, for best results the pressure should be applied by another person who will make his or her essential contribution of energy. Finally, for acupressure to be truly effective, frequent sessions are required for a considerable period, and this may not always be easy to arrange.

However, we have no wish to deny the value of the various systems in use. Their development and their present popularity are important elements in the achievement of a higher standard of health by those who resort to them. They also have the great advantage that those who use them get to know their own bodies better, and such knowledge is very helpful in today's world.

Other traditional methods of stimulation
We shall do no more than give a passing mention here to the process known as the plum tree flower, which consists of gently tapping the skin with a kind of small hammer, the heads of which bristle with fine needles. This technique is used only in special cases or where the insertion of needles would not be tolerated (in young children, for example.)

Cupping, which is still occasionally used in the West, is also employed in the Far East. This stimulotherapy technique has reached a higher degree of refinement there, because the cups (generally made of bamboo and smaller than ours) are even applied to the face. Several other instruments exist for stimulating the skin: rollers mounted on a handle or coins with a hole in the middle which are forcibly thrust flat against the skin.

Modern Methods of Stimulation

The discoveries of modern science have, naturally enough, given rise to new techniques for stimulating the acupuncture points. One of these is Taiki therapy, which will be given a chapter of its own. But first of all let us take a quick look at the other possibilities.

Electropuncture
This method consists of adding electricity to the physical action of the needles. When the needles have been implanted in the skin, the current is switched on. Electrical stimulation then takes the place of manual stimulation with the needles.

Although employed for disorders of certain kinds and also for analgesia (the abolition of sensitivity to pain) by acupuncture this procedure is not recommended for other types of disease (such as heart troubles, for example.)

Electrotherapy
Where this differs from the previous technique is that it relies wholly on electrical stimulation of the points. It was developed as a continuation of the work of Dr Niboyet, who demonstrated the electrical properties of the acupuncture points.

The electrode of the equipment enables the point to be detected in the first place, and is then used to stimulate it electrically. However, as we have already explained, detection of the points by their electrical properties demands particularly stringent test conditions; therefore it is often preferable to locate the points with the help of anatomical plates. The other major drawback of the apparatus is its high cost.

Sonopuncture and laser beams
More recent and less used than electrical stimulation, these are two advanced techniques which are not yet well and truly out of the experimental stage. Sonopuncture stimulates the points by means of sonic vibrations. The vibrations do indeed appear to have some effect on the

points, but the quality of their action is not really known as yet, especially as this must certainly vary with the frequency of the sound waves.

The other technique involves laser beams aimed at the acupuncture points. Here again, much work remains to be done before a proper assessment can be made.

Magnetotherapy and Taiki therapy

We are harking back here to a very old tradition of using magnetism for therapeutic purposes. Yet suddenly it has become right up to date with the advent of very small but powerful magnets.

Modern Explanations of the Action of Stimulotherapies

Confronted by the proven effects of the different types of stimulotherapy on the internal system, modern scientists have endeavoured to find a rational explanation for them. The question is this: how can action on a point in the skin benefit a remote internal organ or the general health of a patient? We state the question in its most general form, since it is not certain that the action of a needle, of pressure, of electricity and of a magnet can be assigned to the same frame of reference. However, as all the explanations put forward at present are no more than working hypotheses, it is too soon to start fitting any particular form of stimulotherapy into a given frame of reference; a better way is to deal with the functioning of stimulotherapies as a whole.

The psychological explanation

This is obviously the first explanation to occur to all the detractors of acupuncture and similar techniques. Their response is simple: the only reason why these therapies work is that the patients believe in them. It is auto-suggestion that does whatever good is done; the beliefs themselves are without foundation.

We hardly think much good would be served by trying to refute this line of reasoning here, even though it is still adopted by some of the old guard in Western medicine who do not want to be disturbed in their cosy world of ideas. The reports are too convincing and too numerous, coming as they do from hundreds of thousands of patients (not counting those in the Far East, of course) and from prestigious international specialists, for this type of explanation to be sustained. The reader who wishes for some proof that is 'above suspicion' is referred to the recent Congress of WHO (the World Health Organization) held in Peking in 1979. *

While on the subject of this explanation of the action of stimulotherapies, we ought perhaps to emphasize the fact that in a unitary concept of the human being, the body and the mind are not independent. What is done to the cutaneous envelope brings into play a mechanism which influences body and mind through body and mind. Far be it from us to belittle the importance of the mental processes; what we do refuse to accept is that stimulotherapy is nothing more than a clever trick that succeeds with the credulous.

Action through neuromediators
The theory that stimulotherapies act through the agency of specific hormones, applies especially to analgesia by acupuncture. It seems that the fact of pricking certain points provokes a more copious secretion of endorphins. These hormones produced in the brain are chemically similar to morphine, and are thought to play a considerable part in the perception of pain. This theory, based on recent work with endomorphins, is partly confirmed by the fact that the injection of a substance antagonistic to morphine (naloxone) suppresses the analgesic effects of acupuncture.

So the action of neuromediators, the secretions of which may well be activated by the pricking of certain points, could be one explanation of acupuncture analgesia. It might then turn out that further effects of acupuncture are brought about through the agency of yet other neuromediators not related to the perception of pain.

* See the WHO magazine *Santé du Monde* for December 1979. (*Santé du Monde*, WHO, avenue Appia, 1211 Geneva 27, Switzerland).

All this is no more than conjecuture, however, and even if a relationship is found between the pricking of a point and the secretion of certain neuromediators, a similar relationship has yet to be established where other methods of cutaneous stimulation are concerned.

Overlap zones in the brain
Dr Amassian * of the University of Baltimore, was the first to reveal the role of the overlapping of body projection zones in the brain. The whole of the human body (and the same sort of thing occurs in animals) is represented in distinct zones of the brain called projections. The size of these projections is not a measure of the size of the organs or other parts of the body represented by them. Thus, the sense organs and the thumb occupy much more space in the brain than do the thigh or the arm. However, the most important fact that Amassian claims to have demonstrated is that these projections very often overlap one another.

This phenomenon is so significant because certain parts of the brain, called overlaps by Amassian, are related to more than one part of the body. If we take, for example, the projection of the hand and the projection of the large intestine, we see that these overlap in the brain. And so a particular point in the hand will be connected with a zone in the brain that is itself conected with the large intestine. It is easy to see how this phenomenon can be used to explain the way in which stimulotherapies work. Pricking or otherwise stimulating some point in the skin presumably sparks off a reaction in this point's projection zone in the brain; if the projection happens to be situated in an overlap, the reaction could well carry through to the other organ or part of the brain represented in that portion of the brain.

This type of explanation, which is not, of course, the last word on the *modus operandi* of acupuncture, since other quite complex laws are involved in Chinese medicine, has the advantage of agreeing with the fact

* Information supplied by J. Borsarello: 'La Médecine chinoise' in *Santé et Médecines naturelles* (Presses médicales européenes, 1976).

that certain points are effective and other are not. Thus those points which project into zones where there are no overlaps may receive local benefit but will never pass that benefit on at a distance.

The action on the tonus of local posture
Here is an interpretation which relies on research carried out in the field of neurophysiology. The hypothesis consists in regarding stimulotherapies as forms of reflexotherapy. That is to say, that treatment of the superficial muscles modifies their tonus locally. This modification is transmitted by specific fibres outside the sensory pathways. The central nervous system, after integrating the modification, starts relaying information that can have repercussions on other regions of the body. * Such a modification, for the most part unconscious, can gain access to the conscious level and become even more effective (as seen, for example, in the conscious physical reactions after a session of acupuncture or massage.)

The interpretation of stimulotherapies as a reflex mode of action has prepared the way for the development of related therapies which do not belong to the Chinese tradition. Reflex massage is a notable example of these.

Conclusion

The above brief account of stimulotherapies as seen through the eyes of Western science, will no doubt have aroused the reader's curiosity concerning traditional Chinese medicine and the way in which this regards acupuncture and its ancillary techniques. Despite considerable efforts that have been made to match acupuncture with bits and pieces taken from our own medical systems, it still turns out that the best way of

---

* This scheme of the 'to-ing' and 'fro-ing' of information has something in common with the theory of overlap zones in the brain, except that in reflexotherapy theory the collecting organ is not the brain but the central nervous system (spinal cord, cerebral trunk, thalamus) and there is no question of localized projection.

using stimulotherapies is to be found in the tradition of the Far East, even if the theoretical reasoning behind it may seem, at first sight, very far removed from our own way of thinking.

4.

THE CHINESE MEDICAL TRADITION

Included in the Chinese medical tradition we find an aggregate of therapies, most of which go back to dim antiquity. Often the therapeutic act itself is performed on the body's cutaneous covering, either by the implantation of a needle (acupuncture), by heat (moxas), or by one of the other methods of stimulation described in the last chapter.

These various therapies are based on complex laws explaining, in terms of energy, Yin-Yang, the meridians, and the elements, what happens when the cutaneous points are stimulated or pharmeceutical substances are ingested. We now propose taking a quick look at these laws, paying special attention to those which have a most direct bearing on stimulotherapies in general and on magnetotherapy in particular.

A Glimpse of Chinese Medical History

It is no easy matter to reconstruct the first empirical advances in the medicine of the Far East, since they took place so far back in the history of China. In short, we may consider that the first therapeutic use of the needle, of heat, and of herbs was made by prehistoric peoples at some time now unknown. According to Dr H. Jarricot and Ming Wong, to whom we are indebted for an 'Essay on the history of Chinese acupuncture' *, acupuncture is most likely to have been developed in eastern China,

* H. Jarricot, Ming Wong, in J.E.H. Niboyet: *Nouveau Traité d'Acupuncture* (Maisonneuve, 1979), pp. 97–186.

moxibustion or the utilization of heat would probably have been suggested by the cold that reigns in the north of China, and the use of medicinal plants seems to have been a conspicious feature of life in the west from time immemorial. All these techniques would have converged on the centre, towards the region of high civilization to be found in the basin of the Yangtsze-Kiang, where a vast syncretism would have come into being.

Be this as it may, it is possible to discern two major contributions to the elaboration of Chinese medicine. One is an experimental knowledge of the virtues of certain therapeutic methods and their probable progressive systematization. For instance, the empirical discovery of the virtues of certain points in the human body, the stimulation of which by pricking or by heat, gave relief, eventually led to descriptions of the meridians linking the points. In the same way, the discovery of the healing properties of certain substances, vegetable and animal, was doubtless improved by using them in combination.

The other contribution was that of the all-embracing concepts developed by Chinese thought, which were applied to ritual, to modes of government and to cosmological speculations. For instance, the terms Yin and Yang seem to have been used about nature in general before they were used in reference to the human organism.

Now, we ought not to imagine that these two contributions were made by distinct professional classes such as our own physicians and philosophers. Over-specialization is the bane of modern times and it is morally certain that at that early epoch the tribal shaman, medicine-man, priest or sage — call him what you will — would take time off from his healing practice for metaphysical speculation.

And so there is little doubt that Chinese medicine, which still has the power to amaze us, was born under the joint influence of experimental discoveries and meditation on the nature of the universe.

From the *Nei Ching* to the Occident
The oldest and most important book on Chinese medicine is the *Huang Ti Nei Ching*. This work stands as the basis of

the whole tradition and there is nothing like it in Western medicine. It could be called the Bible of oriental medicine, in which are enunciated all its essential principles and on which all its practitioners rely. The *Nei Ching* is composed of fragments of varying antiquity, and it is agreed today that it brings together texts ranging from the fifth century BC to some time after the start of the Christian era. The *Nei Ching* falls into two sections: the first is the *Su Wên*, or 'fundamental questions' of the legendary emperor Huang Ti to his physician Ki Bo; and the second is the *Ling Shu*, the classical treatise on acupuncture.

The entire theoretical basis of medicine is already elaborated in the *Su Wên*. We find in it the concept of ch'i — breath or energy – and also the theory of the five elements, of which the first intimations come down to us from the divinatory inscriptions of the thirteenth and fourteenth centuries BC, as well as the concept of the meridians and their location, and most of the other leading principles.

The acupuncture classic, the *Ling Shu*, is more particularly concerned with specifying the course of the meridians and the action of certain points. It also describes the management of the needles and the procedures for utilizing heat in the form of moxas.

Building on the foundations of the totality of the *Nei Ching*, Chinese medicine has not ceased to progress. Let us recall that an imperial college of medicine was founded as long ago as the Tang dynasty (618–907 AD), and that under the Sung, Kin and Yüan dynasties (960–1368 AD) acupuncture and moxibustion entered a golden age. So Chinese medicine was continually enriched over a period of two millenia and had arrived at an extraordinarily high stage of development by the end of that period.

Later on, the traditional system fell into disfavour under the last imperial dynasty (the Ch'ing: 1644–1911) and then under the Kuomintang, but was reinstated with the advent of the New China as proved by this declaration of Mao Tse-tung in 1949: 'The traditional Chinese medicine and pharmacopoeia constitute a rich patrimony. We must do our utmost to explore it and to raise it to a higher level'. Therefore a special effort was made to combine all the fundamental ideas and facts of the tradition and to incorporate contributions from occidental medicine. Among the most spectacular results obtained in the last few years should be mentioned the perfection of analgesia (i.e. anaesthesia without loss of consciousness) by acupuncture and also some of the new stimulotherapies already mentioned.

Concurrently with its evolution in the Far East, certain Western doctors began to take an interest in Chinese medicine from the beginning of the nineteenth century. However, it was not until the return from China of Soulié de Morand, a former French consul in Shanghai, where he was initiated in the art of the needles, that acupuncture was properly presented to the West. Since the publication of his *Précis de la vraie acupuncture chinoise* ('A short account of genuine Chinese acupuncture') in 1934, the number of Western therapeutists practising Chinese medicine has continually increased and a great deal of work has been carried out to try and discover the relationships between occidental concepts and oriental treatments.

Energy

The first and ruling principle of all oriental medicine is that of energy or Ch'i. This term is not peculiar to the vocabulary of medicine but is also a fundamental element in Chinese cosmology. Many orientalists have preferred to translate Ch'i by the word 'breath'. Thus Marcel Granet, in a passage in *La Pensée Chinoise* ('Chinese Thought') devoted to the progression of numbers, tells us that breath is associated with the number 1, because it is 'the unique and primary number, single and total'. * For his part, Henri Maspéro writes,

All things are made of breaths. The nine original breaths were mixed together in the Chaos. When the world was made, the breaths separated. The purest of them ascended to form the heavens; the most gross descended to form the earth. Human bodies are made of these gross breaths; but what gives life and animates them is the original Breath... . †

* M. Granet: *La Pensée Chinoise*, pp.136, 137.
† H. Maspéro: *le Taoïsme et les religions chinoises*.

These few phrases inform us that, to the Chinese mind, Ch'i is first and foremost the cosmic energy that fills the whole universe and that matter is no more than one of its aspects. However, although Ch'i may be the essential principle of the universe, the only way to grasp it effectively is in the phenomena manifesting it. As the *Nei Ching Ling Shu* put it more than two thousand years ago, 'Energy cannot be seen and understood except through its material modifications'. Westerners have concentrated on researching particular aspects of these manifestations of primordial energy, such as mechanical, thermal and electrical energy; but the Chinese have paid a remarkable amount of attention to the manifestations of this energy at the human level, and that is how they have come to develop a medical system founded on an energy-orientated approach to the body's system.

The origins of energy in the human being
The Chinese have never been dualists, and when they tackled the problem of human energies, they did not make a clear-cut separation between matter and energy: 'The living being must not be thought of as matter animated by energy. It is energy that has propelled matter, itself energy, in the direction of vital phenomenon.' (the *Nei Ching Ling Shu*). In fact several levels may be distinguished in manifestations of energy: running all the way from the energy giving rise to matter itself, to the original cosmic energy. And all these mingled manifestations produce life. In order to gain a complete understanding of the human being from the point of view of his energy potential, it is necessary to find out how the latter is constituted. First there is the life force that is transmitted to the child by its parents at the moment of conception. This life force is called the ancestral energy or, to adopt more modern terminology, hereditary energy: it is the equivalent of Maspéro's 'original Breath'.

'And so, at the moment of conception, each individual receives a vital potential proper to himself or herself', if we may adopt the words of A. Faubert. * This energy is

---

* A. Faubert: *Initiation à l'acupuncture traditionelle* (Introduction to traditional acupuncture), (Paris, Belfond, 1974).

given to each of us once and for all. We can modify neither its quality nor its quantity and, ideally, our longevity corresponds to its natural growth curve. We use the word 'ideally' because, in practice, faulty functioning of the energy system (to be described later) will never permit a person to live his ideal curve of life. Therefore the function of 'energy medicine' is to help individuals to achieve the full potential of their life-curves as far as possible. And according to the tradition, this means helping them to live to the age of one hundred or more.

The other main sources of human energy are the energy of the air and the energy supplied by food. The energy of the air corresponds to the oxygen absorbed from the atmosphere; it varies in quantity and quality according to the purity of the atmosphere, and the value derived from it largely depends on the way in which we breathe. The energy stored in our food is extracted from what we eat and drink by several organs (the stomach, spleen and liver).

The energy of air and food are united inside the human body thanks to a system known as the 'triple warmer' or 'tri-heater' (Three Heaters), which amalgamates most of the internal organs. And so these two energies together form the essential energy that, in contrast to the inherited energy, can vary both in quality and in quantity owing to its direct relationship to the properties of the food and air being absorbed, to the individual's breathing habits and to the functioning of the internal organs.

Now, the essential energy and the inherited energy eventually combine, and the resulting energy is that which runs along a particular pathway in the organism (the meridians) to which all the methods of energy stimulation — acupuncture, moxas, massage or Taiki therapy — are applied. Before studying the behaviour of this energy in the human body, that is to say the functioning of the energy system, we must first touch on its essential characteristics: the bipolar manifestation known as Yin–Yang.

Yin and Yang

The ancient Chinese created the words Yin and Yang to

designate two aspects of nature. Yin and Yang are neither forces nor substances *per se* but are rather symbols for the fundamental alternation they observed in the universe. Obviously, it is not possible to offer a precise definition of these two terms, but one or two examples will enable us to grasp their significance fairly quickly.

As a matter of fact, one has only to look at nature to see that it always manifests itself according to two terms. Thus we have day and night, man and woman, dry and moist, heaven and earth, the positive and the negative. Also where there is high there is low; where there is right there is left; where over, under; where convex, concave; where bright, dark, etc. Reality invariably has two aspects, at one and the same time opposed and complementary. Heat, for instance, has no absolute existence but exists in relation to another opposing and complementary aspect, namely cold.

The Chinese, then, have named this bipolarity Yin and Yang. Day, masculinity, dryness, heaven, positivity, brightness, heat are Yang in regard to night, femininity, wetness, earth, negativity, darkness and coldness, which are Yin. Yang is concentration in regard to Yin, which is dispersion.

Nevertheless, the opposition of Yin and Yang must not be regarded as an absolute opposition like that between Good and Evil or between Existence and Non-existence. No, it is an opposition which is both relative and dynamic. It is relative because the Yang exists only in relation to the Yin aspect and vice versa. If, by way of illustration, we take three different temperatures, the intermediate degree will be Yang to the lower degree but Yin to the higher degree. This relativity explains why nothing is totally Yin or totally Yang (there is always a little of Yin in Yang and of Yang in Yin — as perfectly expressed in the celebrated diagram of Tao: the absolute harmony of Yin and Yang). The opposition is dynamic because everything in the universe is in motion, and a Yang phase succeeds a Yin phase as surely as night succeeds day and inspiration succeeds expiration.

Such ideas concerning Yin and Yang impregnate the whole of Chinese thought, and it was inevitable that they should become incorporated in the practice of medicine —

which is the aspect we are now going to explore.

Bipolarity in the human being

The human body and its functioning present themselves under the two aspects of Yang and Yin. Thus each part of the body is Yang in relation to some other part which is Yin to it. The upper part of the body is Yang in regard to the lower part which is Yin; the posterior surface is Yang in regard to the anterior surface which is Yin, the outside of the body is Yang in regard to the inside of the body which is Yin, etc. In the same way, a muscle in contraction is in a Yang phase in regard to its period of relaxation when it is in a Yin phase (systole, Yang; diastole, Yin); the mind is in a Yang phase when awake and in a Yin phase when asleep, etc. Individual personality itself inclines either to Yang or Yin. A thin, nervy person, with a tendency to suffer from insomnia and agitation is more Yang than someone who is fat, flabby, apathetic and somnolent (the latter, if he has all these traits in excess, can be considered as very Yin). Nevertheless, there are always some Yin characteristics tucked away in a Yang personality and vice versa.

Now, besides the fact that the body, the system and the personality manifest themselves in terms of the Yang–Yin bipolarity, we know that energy itself displays the same double aspect. What makes this especially interesting to us is that most diseases appear when there is a lack of balance between the Yang and Yin aspects of energy.

The bipolarity of energy

As we have already seen, Ch'i is first and foremost the original Breath, the cosmic primordial energy, which is fundamentally a unity. However, even at this stage the energy bears within it the latent germs of the two aspects Yang and Yin.

So, as the energy manifests itself, it automatically assumes these two relative opposed and complementary aspects, which are linked in dynamic fashion. (We must beware here of seeing Unity split into the two totally complete and distinct, opposed aspect of Duality, since that mode of thinking is totally alien to the oriental mind.)

Therefore, when it manifests in the human body, energy displays two poles, Yin and Yang; just as a magnet has a south pole and a north pole.

For an individual to enjoy good health, the two poles Yin and Yang of his or her energy must be in the right proportion and in harmony with the environment. If the energy exhibits an excess of Yin or an excess of Yang, the system is unbalanced and illnesses make their appearance. We can distinguish general disorders or local aches and pains which reflect a faulty distribution of the two aspects.

Depression, anxiety, prostration, fear, grief, air-swallowing, fatigue, weakness, anaemia, and low blood pressure, are all manifestations of a general excess of Yin. On the other hand, anger, irritability, agitation, rashness, contractures, cramps, insomnia, thinness, and high blood pressure, are manifestations of a general excess of Yang.

To the two aspects, Yin and Yang, designating the quality of the energy, must be added two other notions characterizing its quantity: the plenitude and the void, or fullness and emptiness. The notion of emptiness signifies the absence of energy; the notion of fullness signifies the superabundance of energy. Obviously, these two terms can find a place in our universal bipolar scheme: the void is Yin, in contrast to the plenitude, which is Yang.

The imbalances characterized by an excess of Yin display symptoms of emptiness, namely dispersion and dilation; and the appropriate therapeutic act aims at concentration and stimulation. The imbalances characterized by an excess of Yang display symptoms of fullness, namely too much concentration and too much tension, and the appropriate therapeutic act aims at dispersion and sedation.

The Circulation of Energy

The bipolarity of energy as it is displayed in human beings is not its sole characteristic. Resulting from a mixture of three different energies (hereditary, of the air and alimentary), on the one hand it subdivides into two energies with different parts to play and on the other hand it travels through the system, following to a precise rhythm the system of the meridians.

Yong and Wei energy
The elaboration and diffusion of energy in the system is carried out by the internal organs, which are grouped in Chinese tradition according to a system called the Tri-heater (Triple Warmer or Three Heaters). It is not necessary here to explore the mechanics of this system; sufficient for us to know that after drawing on the basic energies already described, the Tri-heater diffuses in the body two energies of different types.

One is the energy known as Yong, which is nutritive and deep-seated, and ensures the equilibrium and stability of the energy system as a whole. It is this that circulates in the main meridians.

The other is the energy known as Wei, which is protective and looks after the body's first line of defence against external attack. This energy does not run along the meridians but fills the superficial zones of the body, where it imparts to the skin and muscles their full power to ward off harmful energies trying to invade them from outside.

The existence of Wei energy is fundamental to Taiki therapy since it provides a convincing explanation for part of its action (convincing, we mean, to followers of the Chinese tradition). Thus, it is often a concentration of Wei energy which is answerable for painfulness in certain points situated outside the meridians and responsive to treatment with magnetic pellets. On the other hand, the association of this energy with the muscles gives it a relationship with the psychosomatic role of the muscular carapace, and we shall see later how the magnetic pellets have a psychosomatic part to play when applied to points of tension.

The system of the meridians
The main meridians in which the energy circulates are twelve in number, but as each is symmetrical with regard to the median vertical axis of the human body, there are in all twenty-four meridians answering to twelve different names. It is important to be precise about this because each point described in one part of the body has

its symmetrically placed counterpart in the other part, and it is necessary to treat the two points conjointly.

The meridians are associated with ten organs and two functions recognized by Chinese tradition. That is to say, we have the meridians of the lungs, the large intestines, the stomach, the spleen (with which the pancreas is sometimes associated), the heart, the small intestines, the urinary bladder, the kidneys, the gall bladder, the liver, the tri-heater, and the controller or constrictor of the heart (circulation-sex). The organs usually have a more widely spread function than is attributed to them in the West: thus the large intestine has a connection with inflammatory diseases of the throat and sinuses, while the liver has a connection with sexuality. As for the organic functions, the Tri-heater (or Three Heaters) represents the respiratory, digestive and genito-urinary functions, whereas the controller of the heart represents the sexual organs and the circulation of the blood. Lastly, the characteristic points of a meridian are not necessarily related to the organ after which that meridian is named: on the kidney meridian, for instance, a point can be found which can act on bladder troubles.

The pathway of the meridians commences or terminates in the extremities (the hands and feet), which explains why the points situated in the ends of the limbs (between knee and foot or between elbow and hand) are particularly efficacious: the energy circulates in such a way that it is easier to influence its flow from there.

We should also mention two other special meridians called Marvellous Vessels. These are the Tu-mai and the Jên-mai * situated along the median line of the body (therefore not symmetrical). They both take their origin from a point situated between the anus and the sexual organs and meet again between the nose and the mouth; one runs up the centre of the back and the other up the centre of the front of the body. These meridians contain a number of very effective points and we shall often be indicating in the practical part of this book the points

* Tu-mai means 'governing vessel' and Jên-mai means 'vessel of conception'; terms sometimes used in other books. (Translators note.)

situated in the median line of the abdomen and belonging to the Marvellous Vessel Jên-mai.

The description just given of the system of the meridians is not, however, complete. There are actually eight Marvellous Vessels as well as deep and superficial meridians. Nevertheless, none of them contains other specific points and it is not needful to know them to use the magnetic pellets.

The energy cycles

Energy circulates from one meridian to another in a 24-hour cycle according to an immutable order. This circulation does not imply that all the energy moves along at the same time. What occurs is more like a wave undulating through a closed circuit containing a liquid: the liquid is always present everywhere in the circuit but swells periodically along its whole course. Since there are twelve meridians and the cycle is a daily one of 24 hours, it is normal for each meridian to receive an influx of energy for two hours every day. This daily cycle of energy (in solar hours) is set out below.

Liver meridian	1am to 3am
Lung meridian	3am to 5am
Large Intestines meridian	5am to 7am
Stomach meridian	7am to 9am
Spleen meridian	9am to 11am
Heart meridian	11am to 1pm
Small Intestines meridian	1pm to 3pm
Bladder meridian	3pm to 5pm
Kidney meridian	5pm to 7pm
Heart Constrictor meridian	7pm to 9pm
Three Heaters meridian	9pm to 11pm
Gall Bladder meridian	11pm to 1am

But the circulation of energy is also governed by another rhythm – one that is related to the seasons. Certain organs and the meridians associated with them receive additional energy at set periods of the year. It does not seem necessary to spend time on this, and anyway to do so we should be obliged to go more deeply into the theory of the five elements which has induced the Chinese to include a fifth season in the annual energy cycle.

These daily and seasonal cycles followed by the circulating energy are extremely important for treatments in depth as given by the Chinese medical practitioner. Certain weaknesses in the organs become naturally explicable if these organs are at a trough in the energy cycles. Also, a treatment of the above-mentioned type takes into account the interactions between the organs ruled by the energy cycles.

However, for the sufferer who wants to relieve ordinary aches and pains, it is not indispensable to possess an exact knowledge of all the cyclical laws of energy. The latter are extremely complex and demand thorough study, but the reader should be able to draw several interesting conclusions from their existence. In the first place, they are evidence for the dynamic character of the concept of energy. We are dealing not with a concept of the human being as static but, on the contrary, with the concept of an organism in perpetual motion. In the second place, the relationship between the organism and the universe (indeed their total interdependence) is made evident in the everyday world through these cycles of energy circulating in accordance with cosmic rhythms. For example, the daily cycle is brought into play by the rotation of the earth. In the third place, the energy cycles explain why it is that action on one meridian will affect some other meridian: the disordered state of an organ can be due to blockage in an organ preceding it in the normal run of the energy cycle, and by clearing the blockage in the latter it should be possible to restore the equilibrium of the former.

The Acupunture Points

In setting out from an aspect opposite to that of the previous chapter, we have now worked our way round to the aspect with which that chapter started: the existence in the cutaneous envelope of points possessing therapeutic properties. These points are, so to speak, a concretization of the ideas which have just been expounded; each meridian being laid out along points or 'nodes' of energy the stimulation of which modify, according to strict rules, the energy circulation in general.

Three hundred and sixty-one acupuncture points are counted, distributed unequally along the various meridians; from the meridians of the heart and of the controller of the heart with nine each, to the meridian of the urinary bladder with sixty-seven. In addition there are numerous points outside the meridians. Some of these are in the repertory and their effects are known (e.g. the Yin-t'ang point, situated between the eyes), but there are many others which seem to be suited to particular individuals and symptoms and are not so general in their application. These points are more likely to have to do with the Wei energy, which circulates outside the system of the main meridians. The recognition of such extra-meridional points by Chinese medicine holds a special interest for us, because magnetic pellets are effective on painful points even when these do not lie on the main meridians. The discovery of this type of action was made in the time of the Nei Ching, which recommends: 'the painful places are the points to prick'.

Each of the three hundred and sixty-one points of the twelve main meridians and of the two Marvellous Vessels has a Chinese name and a number in the meridian to which it belongs (it is this number that will be used in the practical part of the book).

The positions of these points were described in the most ancient volumes of Chinese medicine; work carried out in the Far East and in the West during recent decades has simply served to place their positions on a modern anatomical basis. The points given in each meridian fall into several categories. Chief of these are the Shu points situated at the extremities of the limbs, the Luo points which ensure the transfer of energy from one meridian to another, and the source points which regulate the balance of the meridians. The existence of these categories explains why some points are much more important than others. In addition there are several major points with a very powerful action required for many different symptoms. Thus, Stomach thirty-six (Zu San Li), Large Intestines four (Hegu), and conception vessel Jen-mai six and twelve (Qi hai and Zhong Wan), are indicated very frequently as the sites where the magnetic pellets should be placed, just as they are often indicated for treatment by needles or moxas.

The traditional theory of the action of the points

The cutaneous points are the preferred places for intervention in the energy system. By their means, disturbed equilibrium can be corrected in the circulation of energy. And, in the Chinese medical tradition, disturbed equilibrium of this kind is the origin of diseases.

That is to say, disease is assumed to be the symptom of a lack of balance in the energy system. It appears when Yin and Yang are out of proper proportion, when the circulation of energy in the meridians is blocked, when the cycles of energy in the organism are no longer in step with the cosmic cycles. Appropriate action on the point (or points) corresponding to this lack of balance makes it possible for the harmonious circulation of energy to be re-established.

Two main types of action, having an affinity with the universal Yin-Yang bipolarity, have to be considered. One is the dispersing action (Yin); to be applied when there is an energy blockage, an excess of Yang, or over-concentration. The other is the tonifying action (Yang); to be applied when there is a lack of energy, an excess of Yin, too much dispersion. The distinction between the two actions is fundamental in Chinese medical practice but dispersion and tonification must not be compartmentalized too rigidly. Sometimes, in fact, the simple stimulation of a point regulates the energy whatever the type of action employed.

In the case of moxas, for example, the action is considered to be tonifying, but the input of heat is in itself beneficial quite apart from any dispersion or tonification. In the case of magnetic stimulation of the acupuncture points, we are obviously right to think that the north and south poles exert different actions — one dispersing and the other tonifying in character. According to this hypothesis, the north (negative and sedative * pole) would be more dispersing and the south (or positive) pole would be more tonifying. (Remember that, as before, here the north and south poles are British south and north poles respectively.) In practice, however, this scheme appears to be a little too simple; even the application of a bipolar magnetic field, as in the case of certain necklaces made of cylindrical magnets, has the effect of normalizing the energy system. On the other hand, we have already seen that the therapeutic utilization of magnets without reference to the Chinese tradition, is done with the north pole (British south pole) and therefore with a sedative effect. The utilization of polarized magnetic pellets as recommended in the practical section of this book involves placing the north pole (British south pole) in contact with the skin too, and the normalizing effect on the energy system is undeniable.

Apparently the effect of magnetism on the acupuncture points is first and foremost a normalizing one. The employment of the south pole (British north pole) on these points is certainly feasible and would no doubt do good in its own way, but it does present difficulties for the time being and, in our opinion, should be left in the hands of experienced practitioners for further testing.

Whether in fact using magnet therapy or the simulotherapies, the modes of action are numerous and we do not know them all as accurately as we would wish. Therefore, it is very desirable for research to continue into what happens when one or the other magnetic pole is applied to acupuncture points. At present, the application of the north pole (British S.P.) or of bipolar magnets

---

*   'Sedation' and 'tonification' are customarily employed as a pair of terms describing two distinct types of acupuncture action. On the whole, the French author seems to prefer the term 'dispersion' to the term 'sedation'; probably quite rightly, since if the dispersion of a tight knot of energy is the main effect, the sedation or relief from pain will really be no more than a secondary result.   (Translators note.)

works well enough, without giving rise to harmful effects, for it to be recommended as a simple means of stimulation for us by acupuncturists and by the general public. This type of stimulation may be regarded as regulatory, and the disorders that respond to it best are those which experience has led us to present in the practical section of this book.

PRACTICAL GUIDE

5.
MAGNET APPLICATIONS AND TAIKI THERAPY

The magnets intended for use in conjunction with this practical guide are those already referred to as magnetic pellets. Made in Japan, and now on sale in Europe, these magnets vary in their appearance to some extent and also in their size and strength. However, the general pattern (see diagram) displays sufficient specific characteristics for us to be able to envisage a new therapy associating the effects of magnet therapy with the main laws of Chinese acupuncture.

Taiki Therapy

The new method makes use of punctiform and polarized magnetic pellets to stimulate the acupuncture points. In addition to the beneficial effects of magnetic pellets on

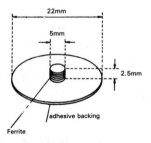

painful regions, as demonstrated by the studies of Nakagawa, this method takes advantage of the laws of acupuncture to act on points situated at a distance from the region touched.

Only the production of magnets powerful enough and

small enough to have a very localized action could have made such a method possible. It is the north pole alone (British S.P.) which is placed next to the skin.

Several levels of interpretation of the action of Taiki therapy are conceivable:

— the effects of magnet therapy;
— the stimulation of specific points defined by Chinese tradition (action on the Wei energy and equilibration of the energy system).

Thinking now of the psychomatic approach to medicine, it is certain that the action of magnets in dealing with physical tensions can prove extremely effective in restoring the balance of the entire being.

This new therapy has the advantage of being directly available for use by the man or woman in the street; whether for the relief of certain minor complaints or as a supplement to other therapies in the case of more serious disorders. Doctors and, in particular, acupuncture practitioners will find in Taiki therapy a far from negligible aid for their treatments in depth, because it can prolong the action on the points between sessions and makes it easier to attend to patients (children and the aged etc.) who do not like the needles or moxas. Lastly, kinesitherapists will be greatly assisted by the magnetic pellets thanks to their action on the muscular tonus (for all strains). In our guide we have distinguished two main levels of use:

— Action on painful areas through the sedative effect of the magnets (the north pole — British S.P.)
— Symptomatic action on local painful points and on points at a distance specified by the laws of acupuncture.

One part has been written particularly with practitioners of Chinese medicine in mind.

In addition to their specific action on the acupuncture points, the presence of magnets on the human body restores the balance of the individual's magnetic field, which thus becomes less vulnerable to external perturbations.

Method of Using the Magnetic Pellets

Here are a few practical rules.

Duration. Generally speaking, the pellets should be worn for three to five days. To leave them on any longer could cause a slight irritation. When the treatment takes some time, the skin must be allowed to rest for two or three days. The period of use can also be shorter and it is proper to remove the pellets as soon as the effect obtained is satisfactory.

Quantity. The number of pellets to be used is very variable — a therapist may prescribe as many as ten to fifteen, but otherwise it is sensible to use no more than two to eight.

Distribution. Except in the case of local aches and pains, for which the magnetic pellets are deposited on a precise region (where there is a sprain, for example), it is preferable to utilize the symmetrical points on each side of the body (in respect of a vertical median plane).

Reutilization. Although the pellets are still magnetized after use, they should be employed no more than twice consecutively and should then be thrown away. So far, we have no rational explanation for this fact, yet they do not have the same therapeutic efficacy after being used but seem to be 'charged' with a noxious energy after treating the points.

Local reaction. Reactions are rare but can take the form of small red spots or eruptions surrounding the pellet. It is then best to leave the skin bare and, if necessary, to disinfect it with diluted tincture of iodine.

Contra-indications. It is necessary to take precautions when there are problems with the skin.

- Avoid using the pellets in the case of cutaneous eruptions. The condition of the skin changes too quickly for one to be able to tell where the rash will appear next.

- Do not place the pellets on areas where the skin is clearly unhealthy. Nevertheless, the pellets will benefit the skin if placed on the appropriate points.

Also, magnetic pellets must not be applied to areas which have been exposed to radiation (as in radiotherapy for cancer) or to areas near metallic protheses. In the latter case the patient's condition could be seriously aggravated. And avoid the proximity of electromagnetic equipment inside or outside the body (hearing aids, pace-makers etc.)

Action on the Painful Zones

The easiest method of using the magnetic pellets, and the one most widely practised, is to apply them to painful zones. That is how members of the general public avail themselves of magnet therapy in Japan, and the statistical studies cited in Chapter 2 refer to treatments of this kind.

The troubles we shall be considering here can have several causes. The two main causes are:

— *a trauma:* sprain, stretched ligament, torn muscle, tennis elbow, certain fractures not placed in plaster (fractured rib, nose, etc.);
— *rheumatism:* lumbago, rheumatism of the hip or shoulder, arthrosis of the cervical column, all joint pains. In general, the pellets are particularly efficacious for chronic rheumatoid inflammations, but afford only slight relief in the case of acute infectious or inflammatory rheumatisms.

Apart from these two main causes there are others of various kinds which give rise to pain in the muscles, joints and tendons. Thus there are complaints due to the weather (chills, the effect of exposure to damp, wind etc.); upset metabolism due to faulty feeding (overindulgence in meat or rich foods which act on the muscles and tendons); poor posture; repercussions on the body of mental tension, which causes the muscles to tighten up through the action of the autonomic nervous system; a state of imbalance in the internal organs which reacts on the external zones.

All these disorders, irrespective of their pathological origin as described above, have some connection with incorrect posture. Thus, considerable benefit can be derived by seeking out points of tension, in order not only to treat these with the magnetic pellets but also to become aware of and to correct any postural problems. All efforts in this direction will be conscious to begin with, but constant repetition will imprint them on the nerve circuits controlling the muscle tone of posture until the improvement is maintained automatically. The fact that magnetic pellets relieve tensions can prove helpful in re-educative therapy of this type.

Placement of the pellets
In each case it is necessary to find the tensest and most painful points in the area to be treated. The best method is to pass the thumb over the painful zone while exerting moderate pressure. The points that seem to be harder, stiffer and more sore than the surrounding ones, are the ones where the pellets should be placed. Usually they will turn out to be the well-known acupuncture points on the meridians.

In the following pages the reader will find a series of plates to help in locating the points. The various aches and pains are considered here simply from a local point of view, without reference to their origin; but, of course, each pain is individual and other points than those indicated can be discovered.

For the most part, there will be no need to place the pellets on each side of the body, except when the points are close to the median regions.

Finally, many of the troubles described are chronic, and one should not hesitate to use the magnetic pellets regularly and repeatedly, while always allowing a break of two or three days between successive applications of the pellets to the same point.

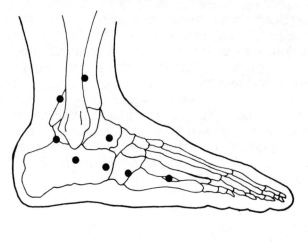

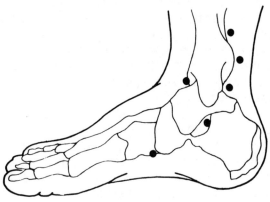

ANKLE PAIN

This is generally the result of a sprain. According to the way the ankle was twisted, the painful points will be situated mainly on either the outside or the inside of the ankle.

It is nearly always necessary to treat one or other of two points situated either on the external malleolus (Urinary Bladder 62) or on the internal malleolus (Kidney 6). These two are prime energy points.

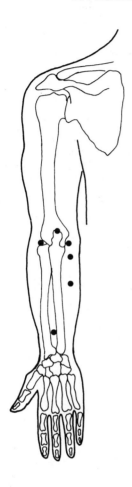
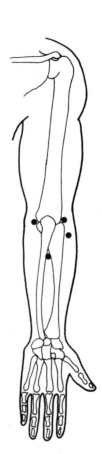

ELBOW PAIN

There are several very important energy points which
have to be tested (see illustration). Look for them on the
anterior surface of the forearm near the elbow and on the
posterior surface near the wrist. Also try to find the
sensitive points on the nape of the neck and along the
upper dorsal column.

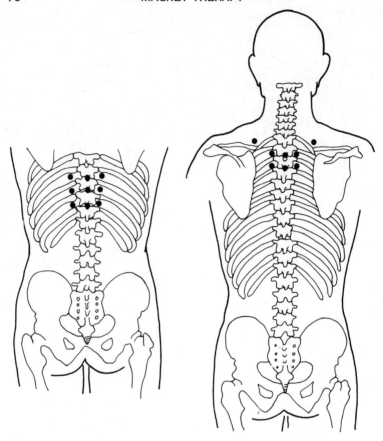

BACKACHE

The painful points are usually situated at two fingers' breadth on each side of the spine. These are the points of the urinary bladder meridian corresponding to the internal organs.

The magnetic pellets can also be placed where two vertebrae meet, either when there is definite pain there, or when one vertebral process is not in alïgnment with the others or does not seem to stand out as well as the vertebral processes do on the back. The pellets correct the tonus of the paravertebral muscles and help the spine to return to true.

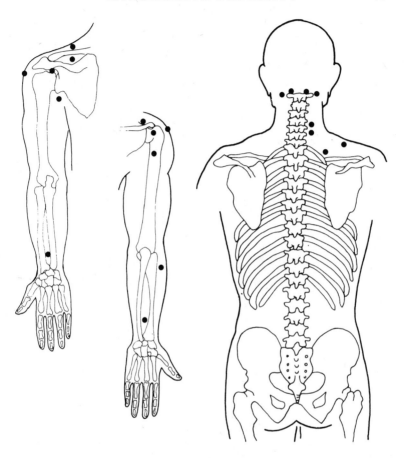

SHOULDER PAIN

The points to treat are situated on the same side as the pain. Note the movement which does most to aggravate the pain. For instance, if it is a forward movement of the arm, a magnetic pellet should be applied to the anterior surface.

Feel for sore points in the nape of the neck, along the upper dorsal column and down the arms to well below the elbows. The diagram shows certain potentially painful points at quite some distance from the shoulder, and these may need treatment.

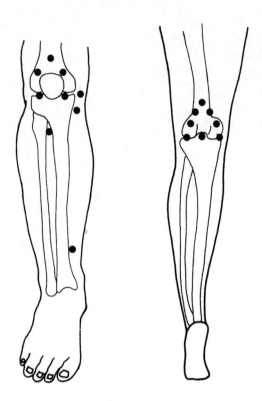

PAIN IN THE KNEES

Generally speaking, this type of pain is chronic and the treatment can be repeated.

There are some very important acupuncture points in this region (shown in the illustration); these should always be treated if they are painful, although it goes without saying that treatment ought to be given to any painful point wherever it is.

Knee pain often has some connection with the sacro-lumbar region and the points in this region ought therefore to be tested (both on the same side as the knee in question and on the oppostie side to it) to determine whether or not they are painful on pressure; if so, they should be treated.

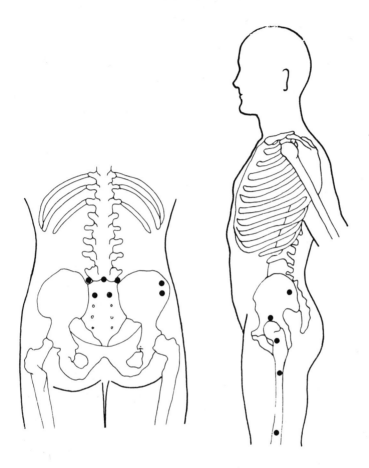

HIP PAIN

The points requiring treatment are chiefly near the hip joint (the external or posterior surface), on the buttocks, and also along the thigh. It is important to locate tense zones on the latter which often correspond to the gall bladder meridian on the outer surface and, more rarely, to the stomach meridian on the anterior surface.

Magnetic pellets may also be required on points in the back around the sacrum; in which case they should be placed on both sides of the spine even if the pain is in one hip only.

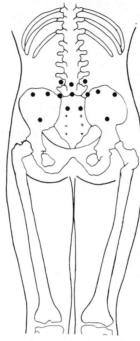

LUMBAR PAIN

We include in this term pains in the loins, lumbago, a strained back, and other minor pains. Usually, the ground has been prepared by an arthritic tendency and the trouble is sparked off by an awkward movement of the body or by some climatic influence (cold or damp, say).

The points to treat are situated mainly in the region of the lumbar spinal column and of the sacrum, since the pain often appears when the disc between the last lumbar vertebra and the sacrum is in poor condition.

It is possible to place the magnetic pellets on the vertebral column, but always at the junction between two vertebrae. Very often it is necessary to locate the pellets on each side of the column in the painful region — not only where the suffering is greatest but on any tense points higher up.

The buttocks should be gently prodded to find painful points.

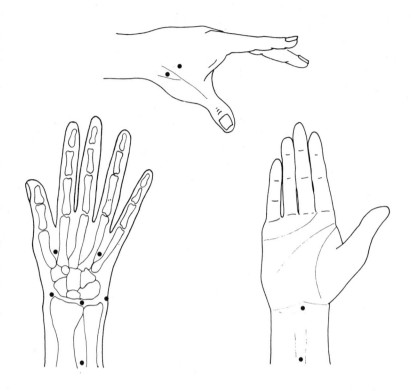

PAIN IN THE HAND AND WRIST

Proceed as usual to look for painful points. However, as it is difficult to place magnetic pellets on the fingers, the points illustrated in the diagrams should be treated according to their sensitivity. These are found: on the back of the wrist (Three Heaters 5); on the back of the hand between the metacarpals of the thumb and the index finger (Large Intestine 4); where the prolongation of the thumb articulates with the wrist (Large Intestines 5). In the case of Dupuytren's disease — retraction of the tendons of the hand on the anterior surface — magnetic pellets can be a considerable help when placed on the anterior surface of the wrist joint on the median line between the tendons (Heart Constrictor 7) and at three fingers' breadths along the forearm on the same line (Heart Constrictor 6).

PAIN IN THE NAPE OF THE NECK

This trouble chiefly arises from a stiff neck or from cervical arthrosis, but can also be due to the presence of tensions caused by digestive disturbances (liver, gall bladder), or by holding the head incorrectly.

Sore points will be found either along the cervical column, in which case the magnetic pellets are placed between two vertebrae, or else at the base of the cranium and on the front or back of the neck (where unfortunately the hair sometimes gets in the way.)

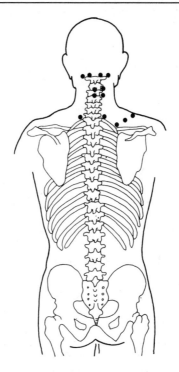

PAIN IN THE THORAX

The pellets are particularly useful for intercostal neuralgia. In general, although the painful points vary from person to person, they are very easy to find (these are extra-meridional points).

Symptomatic Action

In this section we shall be considering the effects of magnetic pellets on certain well-known disorders. Some of them can be treated without calling in a doctor provided the pellets are used in the very early stages (in the case of a sore throat, for instance). Other disorders do call for qualified help but the magnetic pellets make a good form of supplementary therapy (in asthma or obesity, say), or afford temporary relief (as when the patient is waiting for the dentist to treat a toothache). In each case, it is important to observe carefully how the symptoms are developing and to consult a medical practitioner when necessary.

All the ailments are usually projections on the body near the affected zone. We invariably indicate the most important points to treat locally, but others not mentioned may be painful and it will then be necessary to give these priority. We also show the main energy points acting at a distance on the disorder in question.

We deal with the points as falling in two groups. Those underlined are the most important. Nevertheless, this does not imply that the others are negligible. In fact, the reader is advised to discover the points that will do him or her most good.

To locate the points, refer to the anatomical description and to the illustrations. The word 'pouce' is a technical term and means the distance between the two creases of the second phalange of the middle finger. Three fingers' breadth is roughly equal to two pouces. The black point in the diagram is the most important point.

AIR SWALLOWING

Points to treat locally on the chest and abdomen:

Jên-mai 16:   in the median line, one pouce below the base of the sternum.

Jên-mai 12:   half-way between the navel and the base of the sternum

Kidney 21:   six pouces above the navel, level with the union of the sixth and seventh ribs,

one fingers' breadth from the median
line.

Jên-mai 21: in the centre of the sternal fork, level
with the bone.

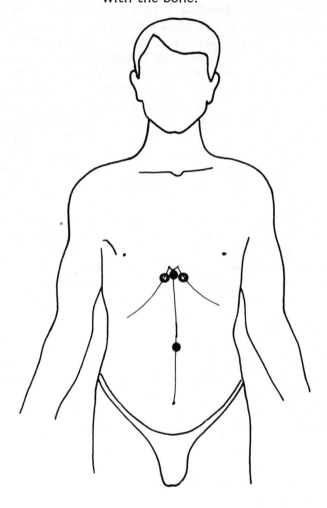

On the back:
*Urinary
Bladder 21:* on the horizontal line between the
twelfth dorsal vertebra and the first
lumbar vertebra, one and half pouces
from the median line.

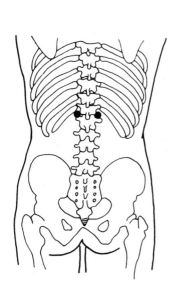
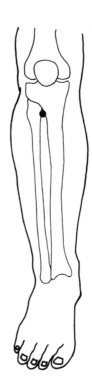

Remote point:
Stomach 36:   four fingers' breadth below the kneecap and two fingers' breadth to the outside of the tibial crest.

EMACIATION

The treatment has to be repeated over a long period of time. It complements other forms of treatment.

Jên-mai 6:   median line, one and a quarter pouces below the navel.

Jên-mai 12:   half-way between the navel and the base of the sternum.

Stomach 25:   horizontal with the navel and two pouces from the median line.

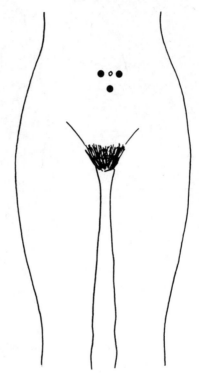

Spleen 4:   on the inside edge of the foot, just
                      under the metatarsal-cuneiform
                      articulation.

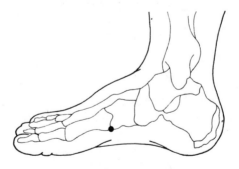

Urinary   on the horizontal line passing between
Bladder 13:   the third and fourth dorsal vertebrae,
                      one and a half pouces from the median
                      line.

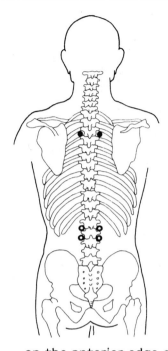

Gall Bladder 39:	on the anterior edge of the fibula, two fingers' breadth above the external malleolus.
Urinary Bladder 22:	on the line passing between the first and second lumbar vertebrae, one and a half pouces from the median line.
Urinary Bladder 23:	on the horizontal passing between the second and third lumbar vertebrae, one and a half pouces from the median line.

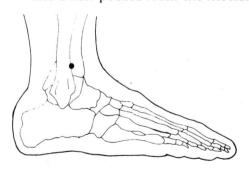

ASTHMA

Points to treat locally:

Jên-mai 17:   on the median line of the body under the relief joining the fourth ribs.

Jên mai 21:   in the centre of the sternal fork, level with the bone.

Urinary Bladder 11:   horizontal with the apophysis of the first dorsal vertebra, one and a half pouces from the median line.

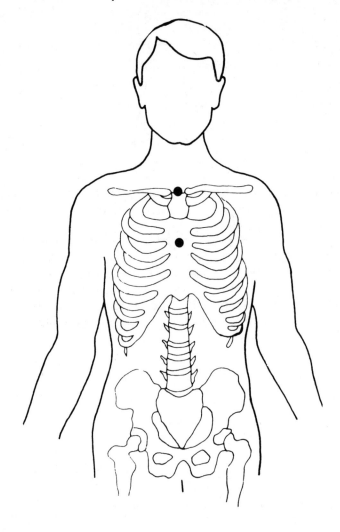

Urinary
  Bladder 13:   on the horizontal separating the third and fourth dorsal vertebrae, one and a half pouces from the median line.

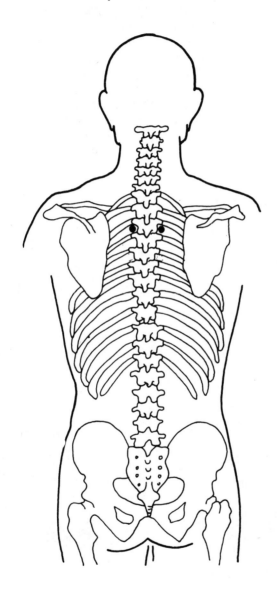

Remote points:
Stomach 36:   four fingers' breadth under the kneecap and two fingers' breadth outside the tibial crest.
Lung 5:   level with the elbow fold on the external border of the tendon.

If the asthma attack is caused by something that has been eaten, you may also treat:
Stomach 40:   slightly more than half-way up the external surface of the leg, about one pouce outside the tibial crest.

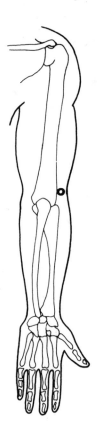 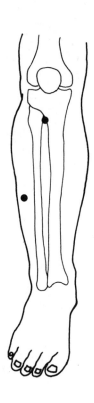

BUZZING IN THE EARS

Points to treat locally:

Small
Intestines 19: in front of the ear-lobe and behind the tempero-maxillary articulation.

Three Heaters
17: in the hollow formed between the lobule of the auricle and the mastoid bone when the mouth is opened.

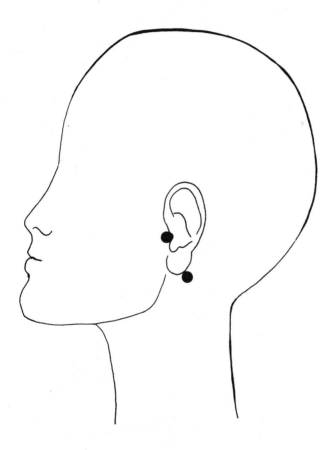

Gall Bladder
20: one pouce from the occiput and two and a half fingers' breadth from the median line.

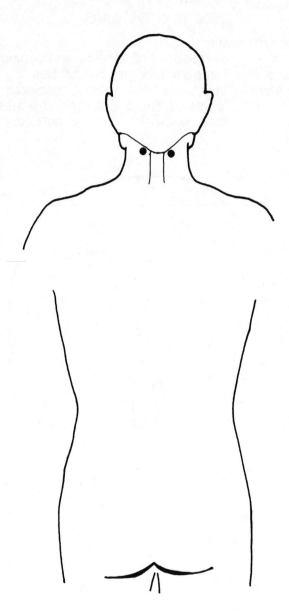

Remote point:
Three Heaters
5: two pouces from the crease of the wrist, between the radius and the ulna, on the dorsal surface of the forearm.

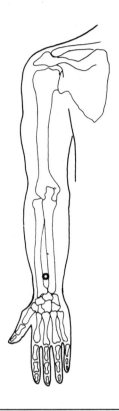

CONSTIPATION

Points to be treated locally on the abdomen:

Stomach 25:   horizontal with the navel, two pouces from the median line.

Jên-mai 5:   on the median line, two pouces under the navel.

Points to be treated locally on the back:

Urinary Bladder 28:   at the height of the second sacral foramen, some four fingers' breadth from the median line.

Urinary Bladder 25:   on the horizontal line between the fourth and fifth lumbar vertebrae, one and a half pouces from the median line.

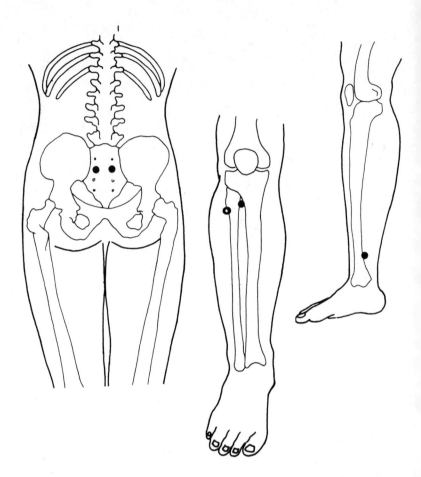

Remote points:

Stomach 36: four fingers' breadth below the kneecap and two fingers' breadth to the outside of the tibial crest.

Spleen 6: on the inside of the leg, against the posterior border of the tibia, four fingers' breadth above the internal malleolus (do not use during pregnancy).

Gall Bladder 34: on the outside of the leg, in the hollow under the head of the fibula.

DIARRHOEA

Points to be treated locally:

Jên-mai 12:   half-way between the navel and the base of the sternum.

Jên-mai 11:   on the median line, three fingers' breadth above the navel.

Stomach 25:   horizontal with the navel, two pouces from the median line.

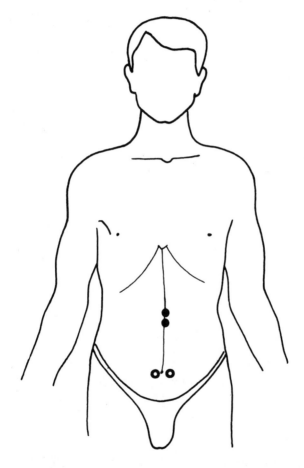

Remote points:

Stomach 36:   four fingers' breadth below the kneecap and two fingers' breadth on the outside of the tibial crest.

Kidney 7:   on the inside of the leg, three fingers' breadth above the internal malleolus and one and a half pouces behind the border of the tibia.

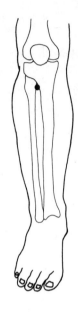 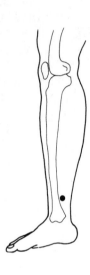

HEAVY OR SLOW DIGESTION

Points to be treated locally:

Jên-mai 12:   half-way between the navel and the base of the sternum.

Kidney 21:   six pouces above the navel, level with the union of the sixth and seventh ribs, one fingers' breadth from the median line.

Also to be considered for treatment are all the painful points of the vessel of conception, Jên-mai, which runs along the median line of the front of the body; in particular those points situated between the navel and the sternum.

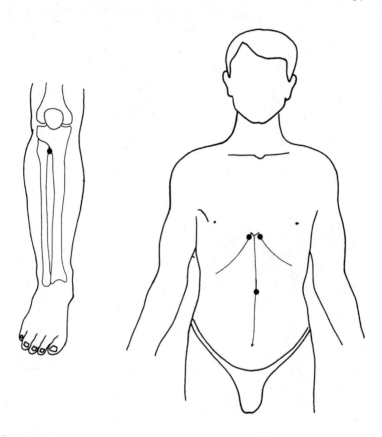

Remote points:

Stomach 36:   four fingers' breadth under the kneecap and two fingers' breadth on the outside of the tibial crest.

Spleen 4:   on the inside of the foot, just under the metatarso-cuneiform articulation.

Large Intestine 4:   in the angle formed by the first two metacarpals.

You can also choose the painful points from among Urinary Bladder 18, 19, 20 and 21: these are situated on the back, one and a half pouces from the median line and on the horizontal between the ninth and tenth, tenth and eleventh, and eleventh and twelfth dorsal vertebrae, and between the twelfth dorsal and the first lumbar vertebrae.

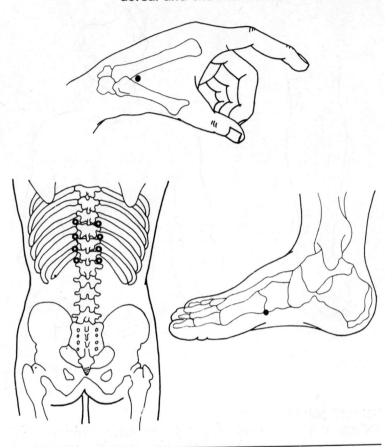

ABDOMINAL PAIN, DISTENSION OF THE STOMACH

Points to treat locally on the abdomen:

Jên-mai 5:   on the median line, two pouces below the navel.

Stomach 25:   horizontal with the navel, two pouces from the median line.

The painful points situated below Stomach 25 (Stomach 27, 28, 29).

On the back:

Urinary Bladder 25:	on the horizontal between the fourth and fifth lumbar vertebrae, one and a half pouces from the median line.
Urinary Bladder 29:	at the height of the third sacral foramen on the sacral border, four fingers' breadth from the median line.

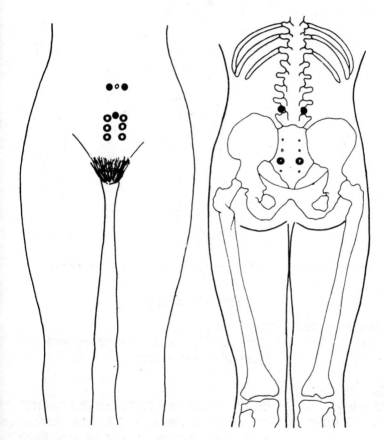

Remote points:

Stomach 36:	four fingers' breadth below the kneecap, two fingers' breadth outside the iliac crest.
Stomach 37:	eight fingers' breadth below the kneecap and two fingers' breadth outside the tibial crest.

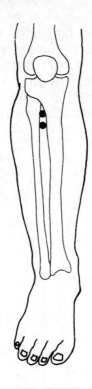

STOMACH ACHE

Points to treat locally on the abdomen:
Jên-mai 12:   half-way between the navel and the
                       base of the sternum.

On the back:
Urinary   on the horizontal between the twelfth
  Bladder 21:   dorsal vertebra and the first lumbar
                       vertebra, one and a half pouces from
                       the median line.
Urinary   on the horizontal between the eleventh
  Bladder 20:   and twelfth dorsal vertebrae, one and a
                       half pouces from the median line.
Urinary   on the horizontal between the ninth
  Bladder 18:   and tenth dorsal vertebrae, one and a
                       half pouces from the median line.

Remote point:
Stomach 36:   four fingers' breadth below the
kneecap and two fingers' breadth
outside the tibial crest.

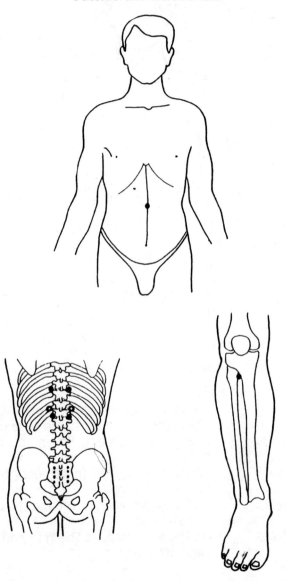

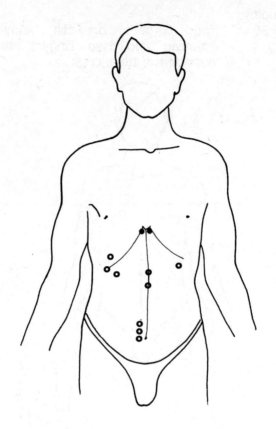

PAIN IN THE GALL BLADDER

Points to treat locally:

Kidney 21:   six pouces below the navel, level with the union of the sixth and seventh ribs, one fingers' breadth from the median line.

Jên-mai 13:   on the median line, five fingers' breadth above the navel.

Jên-mai 12:   half-way between navel and the base of the sternum.

Liver 13:   on the abdomen, at the free end of the eleventh rib.

Also any painful points situated under the ribs on the right: Stomach 23, 24, 25; Gall Bladder 24; Spleen 16.

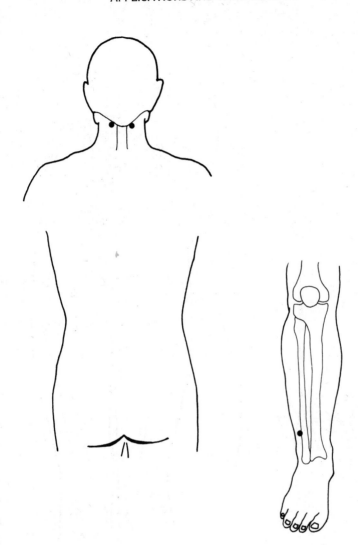

Remote points:

Gall Bladder 37: in the lower third on the outside of the leg, five pouces above the external malleolus.

Gall Bladder 20: one pouce below the occiput and two fingers' breadth from the median line.

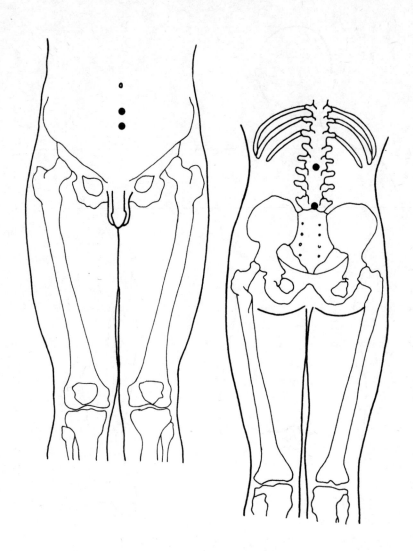

ENURESIS (BED-WETTING)

Points to be treated locally, on the abdomen:

Jên-mai 6:   median line, about one and a quarter pouces below the navel.

Jên-mai 4:   median line, three pouces below the navel.

Points on the back:

Tu-mai 3:	median line, below the spinous process of the fifth lumbar vertebra.
Tu-mai 4:	median line, below the spinous process of the second lumbar vertebra.

Remote points:

Stomach 36:	four fingers' breadth below the kneecap, and two fingers' breadth outside the tibial crest.
Small Intestines 5:	on the outside edge of the wrist, in the hollow level with the main crease of the wrist (racette).

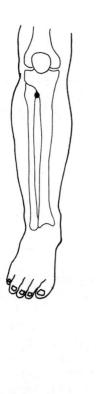
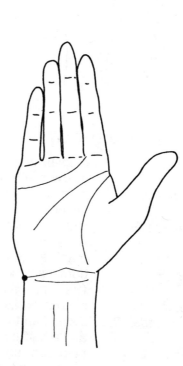

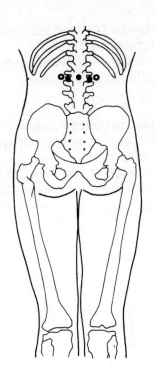 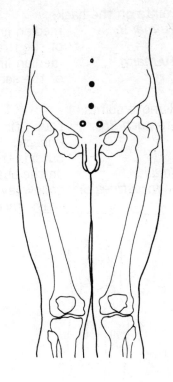

FRIGIDITY — IMPOTENCE

Jên-mai 6:	median line, one and a quarter pouces below the navel.
Jên-mai 4:	median line, three pouces below the navel.
Stomach 36:	four fingers' breadth below the kneecap, and two fingers' breadth outside the tibial crest.
Liver 3:	dorsal surface of the foot, between the first and second metatarsals.
Urinary Bladder 23:	on the horizontal passing between the second and third lumbar vertebrae, one and a half pouces from the median line.
Tu-mai 4:	below the spinous process of the second lumbar vertebra.
Stomach 29:	one fingers' breadth above the pubis and two pouces from the median line.

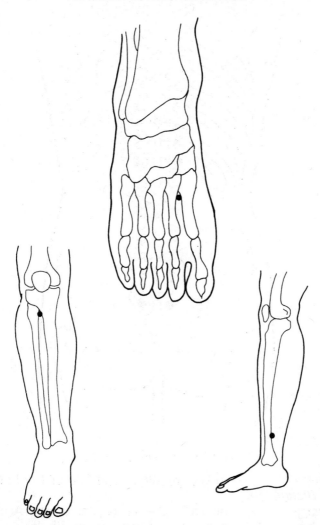

Urinary *Bladder 47:*	on the horizontal passing through the second and third lumbar vertebrae, four pouces from the median line.
Spleen 6:	on the inside of the leg, against the posterior border of the tibia, four fingers' breadth above the internal malleolus.

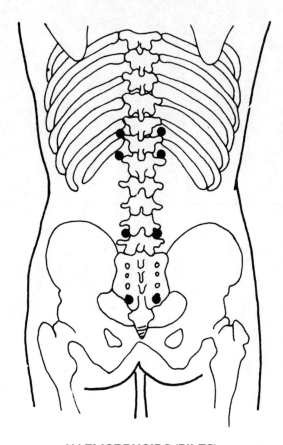

HAEMORRHOIDS (PILES)

Urinary Bladder 54:	in the middle of the fold of the knee.
Urinary Bladder 58:	on the external border of the Achilles tendon, half-way up the fibula.
Urinary Bladder 30:	at the lower angle of the sacrum and of the insertion of the gluteus maximum.
Urinary Bladder 20:	on the horizontal between the eleventh and twelfth dorsal vertebrae, one and a half pouces from the median line.
Urinary Bladder 21:	on the horizontal passing between the twelfth dorsal vertebra and the first lumbar vertebra, one and a half pouces from the median line.

Urinary
  Bladder 25:   on the horizontal passing between the fourth and fifth lumbar vertebrae, one and a half pouces from the median line.

Stomach 36:   four fingers' breadth below the kneecap and two fingers' breadth outside the tibial crest.

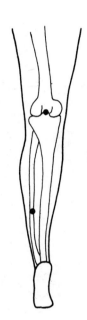
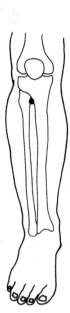

INFLAMMATION OF THE BLADDER AND URETER

Points to treat locally on the abdomen:
Jên-mai 3:   median line, four pouces below the navel.

On the back:
Urinary
  Bladder 28:   at the height of the second sacral foramen, about four fingers' breadth from the median line.

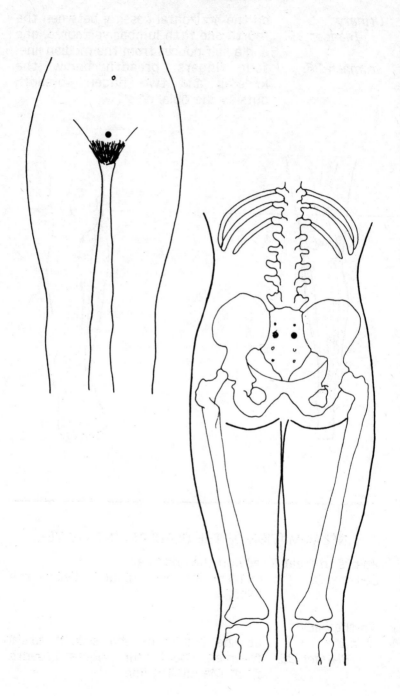

Remote points:

Spleen 6:	on the inside of the leg, against the posterior border of the tibia, four fingers' breadth above the internal malleolus (not to be used during pregnancy).
Spleen 9:	on the inner side of the knee on the edge of the angle formed by the head and body of the tibia.
Large Intestine 11:	just above the outside extremity of the elbow fold.

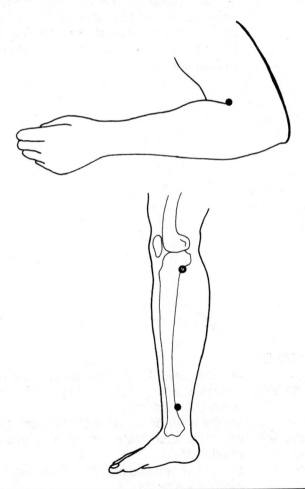

LEG WEAKNESS

Points to treat locally:

Spleen 6:   on the inside of the leg, against the posterior border of the tibia, four fingers' breadth above the internal malleolus (not to be used during pregnancy).

Spleen 9:   on the inner side of the knee on the edge of the angle formed by the head and body of the tibia.

Kidney 9:   on the inside of the leg, two fingers' breadth behind the ridge of the tibia, a little more than half-way up the leg (about six pouces above the internal malleolus).

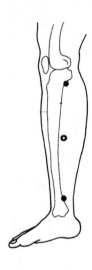

Remote points:

Urinary
  Bladder 28:   at the height of the second sacral foramen about four fingers' breadth from the median line.

Urinary
  Bladder 30:   on the inferior angle of the sacrum and of the insertion of the gluteus maximum.

Tu-mai 3:   below the spinous process of the second lumbar vertebra.

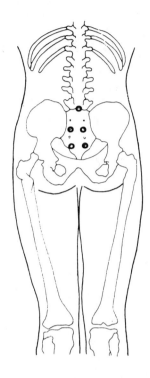

SORE THROAT

Points to treat locally:

Jên-mai 21:   in the middle of the sternal fork, flush with the bone.

Stomach 9:   on the side of the neck, on the course of the carotid artery.

Treat the other painful points on the throat. Pellets can also be placed on any swollen glands. The effect varies considerably from individual to individual: some people find the pellets very effective: others cannot tolerate them — in which case it is sufficient to remove the pellets.

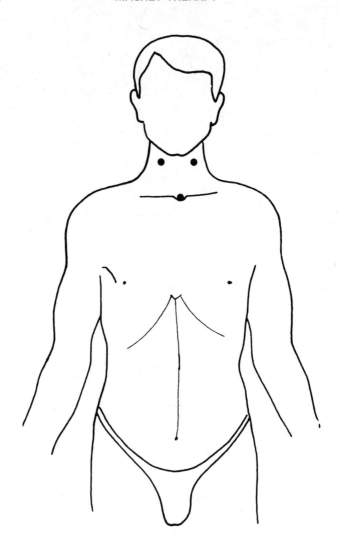

Remote points:

Large Intestine 4:	in the angle formed by the first two metacarpals.
Gall Bladder 20:	one pouce below the occiput and two fingers' breadth from the median line.
Gall Bladder 39:	on the anterior border of the fibula, two fingers' breadth from the external malleolus.

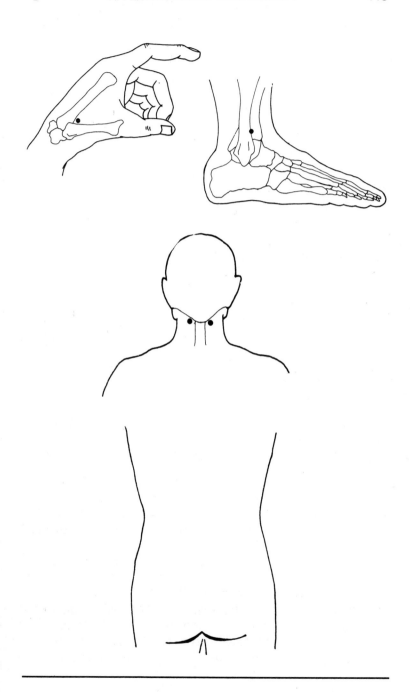

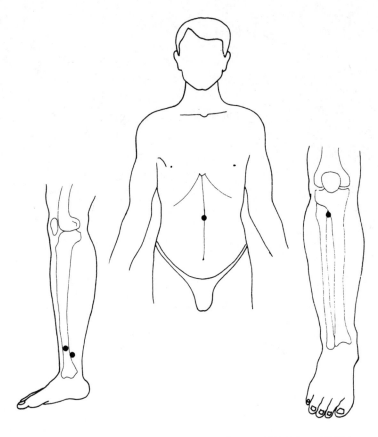

SKIN DISEASES (ACNE, PIMPLES, WARTS, ETC.)

Jên-mai 12:   half-way between the navel and the base of the sternum.

Stomach 36:   four fingers' breadth below the kneecap and two fingers' breadth outside the tibial crest.

Liver 5:   on the inside of the leg, five pouces above the internal malleolus on the internal surface of the tibia.

Spleen 6:   on the inside of the leg, against the posterior border of the tibia, four fingers' breadth above the internal malleolus (do not use during pregnancy).

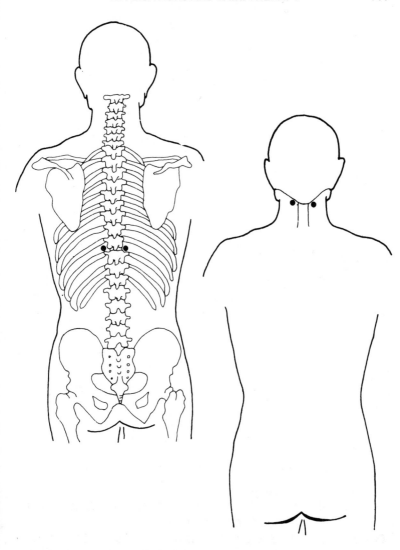

Urinary   on the horizontal between the ninth
Bladder 18:   and tenth dorsal vertebrae, one and a
                     half pouces from the median line.
Gall Bladder one pouce below the occiput and two
20:   and a half fingers' breadth from the
                     median line.

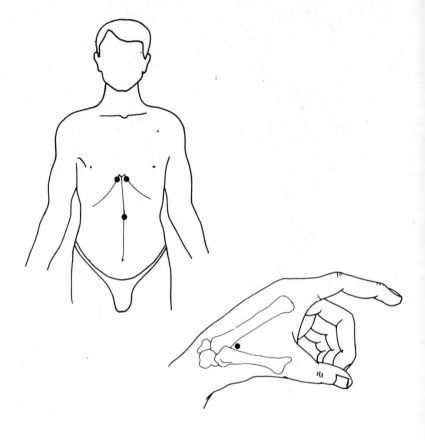

NAUSEA, TRAVEL SICKNESS

Points to treat locally:

Jên-mai 12:   half-way between the navel and the base of the sternum.

Kidney 21:   six pouces above the navel, level with the union of the sixth and seventh ribs, and one fingers' breadth from the median line.

Remote point:

Large Intestine 4:   in the angle formed by the two metacarpals.

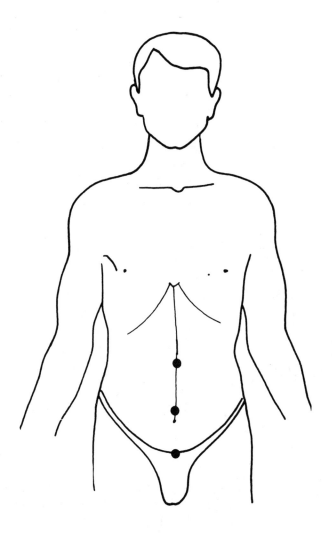

OBESITY

This treatment has to be repeated over a long stretch of
time. It complements other treatments.

Jên-mai 4:	median line, three pouces below the navel.
Jên-mai 9:	median line, one pouce above the navel.
Jên-mai 12:	half-way between the navel and the base of the sternum.

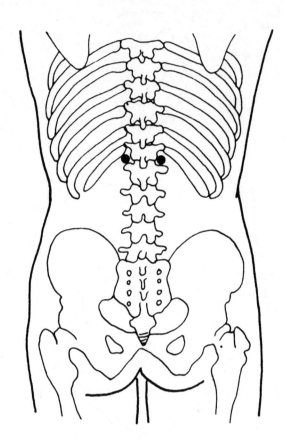

Jên-mai 21:   on the horizontal between the twelfth dorsal and the first lumbar vertebra, one and a half pouces from the median line.

Spleen 6:   on the inside of the leg, against the posterior border of the tibia, four fingers' breadth above the internal malleolus (do not use during pregnancy).

Stomach 36:   four fingers' breadth below the kneecap, and two fingers' breadth outside the tibial crest.

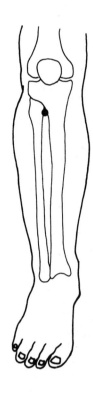
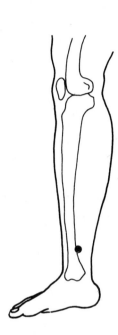

PALPITATION, CARDIAC SPASMS

Points to treat locally:

Jên-mai 14:	median line, two pouces below the base of the sternum.
Jên-mai 15:	median line, one pouce below the base of the sternum.
Kidney 24:	between the third and fourth ribs, two pouces from the median line.
Kidney 25:	between the third and second ribs, two pouces from the median line.

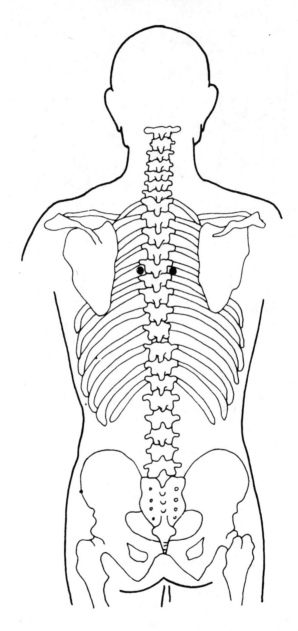

Bladder 15:   on the horizontal passing between the
fifth and sixth dorsal vertebrae, one
and a half pouces from the median line.

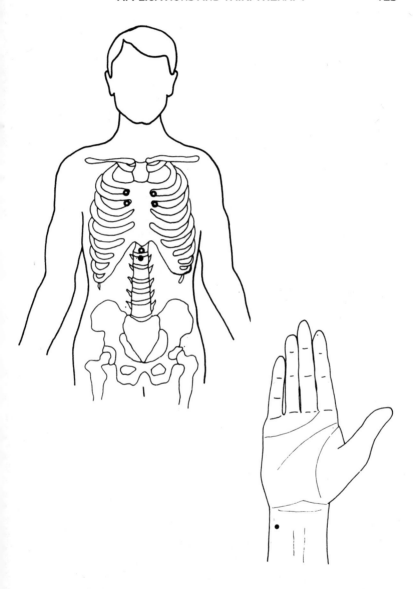

Remote point:
Heart 5:   on the anterior surface of the wrist, in
                             the radical groove, opposite the styloid
                             process.

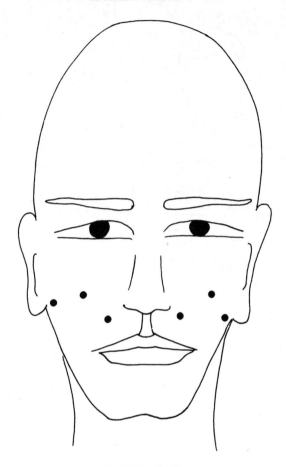

TOOTHACHE

Points to treat locally (according to the place of the trouble):

Large
  Intestines 20:   half a fingers' breadth from the wing of the nose, slightly above the horizontal line passing under the nose.

Small
  Intestines 18:   at the intersection of the external angle of the eye and of a horizontal passing the lower border of the nose.

Stomach 3:   between the angle of the inferior maxillary and the ear lobe (in the hollow formed when the mouth is opened).

Remote points:

Large Intestines 4:	in the angle formed by the first two metacarpals.

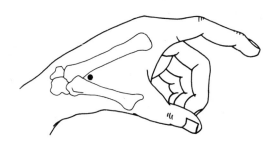

Stomach 44:	half a pouce behind the angle formed by the second and third toes, rather on the side of the second toe.

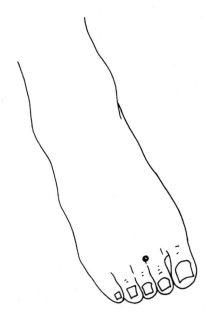

Three Heaters 5:	two pouces from the fold of the wrist (racette) between ulna and radius, on the dorsal surface of the forearm.

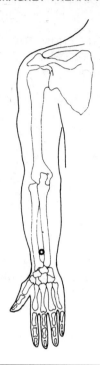

COLD IN THE HEAD — SINUSITIS

Points to treat locally:

Large Intenstines 20:	half a fingers' breadth from the wing of the nose, a little above the horizontal passing under the nose.
Bladder 2:	at the end of the brow ridge next to the nose under the eyebrows, half a fingers' breadth from the median line.
Yin-t'ang point:	an extra-meridional point between the eyebrows on the median line.

You can also treat the extra-meridional points situated near the nose. With any of these points on the face, it is sufficient to leave the pellets in place during the night or when it is possible to stay at home.

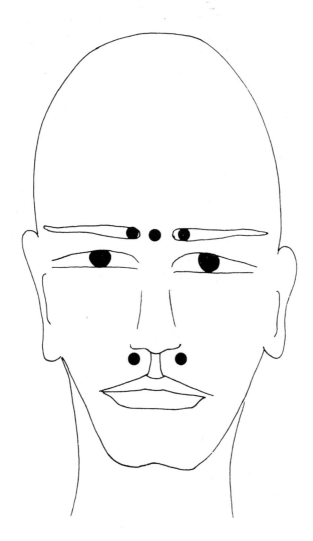

Remote points:
Bladder 12:   one and a half pouces from the spinal
                    column, on the horizontal line separat-
                    ing the second and third dorsal
                    vertebrae.
Tu-mai 13:   on the body's median line between the
                    seventh cervical and first dorsal
                    vertebrae.

Gall Bladder 20:	one pouce below the occiput and two fingers' breadth from the median line.
Large Intestine 4:	in the angle formed by the first two metacarpals.

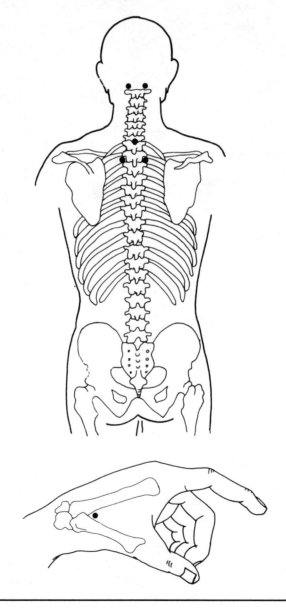

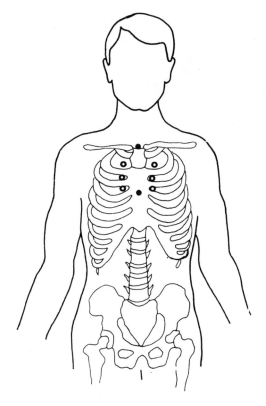

COUGH

Points to treat locally on the chest:

Jên-mai 21: in the centre of the sternal fork, flush with the bone.

Jên-mai 17: median line of the body, below the relief joining the fourth ribs.

Jên-mai 18: median line of the body, below the relief joining the third ribs.

Kidney 24: between the fourth and third ribs, about two pouces from the median line.

Kidney 25: between the third and second ribs, about two pouces from the median line.

Kidney 26: between the second and third ribs, about two pouces from the median line.

See if any of the last-mentioned kidney meridian points are painful and, if so, include them in the treatment.

Points on the back:

Urinary   one and a half pouces from the spinal
  Bladder 12:   column, on the horizontal line separat-
               ing the second and third dorsal
               vertebrae.

Tu-mai 13:   on the median line of the body between
               the seventh cervical and the first dorsal
               vertebrae.

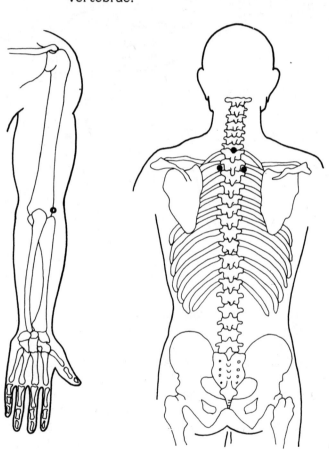

Remote point:

Lung 5:   level with the elbow fold on the
               external border of the tendon.

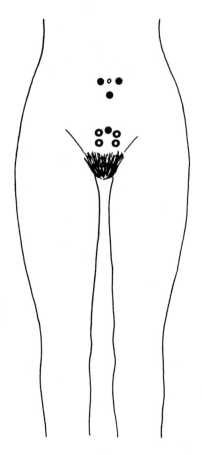

MENSTRUAL DISORDERS (PAIN, IRREGULAR PERIODS)

Points to treat locally on the abdomen:

Jên-mai 6:   median line, about one and a quarter pouces below the navel.

Jên-mai 4:   median line, three pouces below the navel.

Stomach 25:   horizontal with the navel, two pouces from the median line.

Stomach 29:   one fingers' breadth above the pubis and two pouces from the median line.

Stomach 28:   three pouces below the horizontal line passing through the navel, and two pouces from the median line.

Points on the back:

Urinary   at the height of the second sacral
  Bladder 28:   foramen, about four fingers' breadth
                 from the median line.
Urinary   in the inferior angle of the sacrum and
  Bladder 30:   of the insertion of the gluteus
                 maximum.

Remote points:

Spleen 6:   on the internal surface of the leg,
                 against the posterior border of the
                 tibia, four fingers' breadth above the
                 internal malleolus.
Spleen 9:   on the internal surface of the knee, on
                 the edge of the angle formed by the
                 head and body of the tibia.

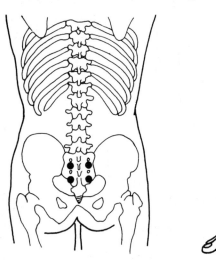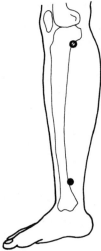

DEFECTIVE EYESIGHT

Points to treat locally (the pellets being worn during the
night, say):

Urinary   at the end of the superciliary arch
  Bladder 2:   under eyebrows, one fingers' breadth
                 from the median line.
Three Heaters   at the tip of the eyebrow, on the outer
      23:   border of the orbit.

Gall Bladder 13:	on the vertical passing through the outer extremitiy of the eyebrow, half a pouce below the hairline.

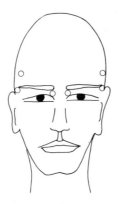

Remote points:

Large Intestines 4:	in the angle formed by the first two metacarpals.
Gall Bladder 20:	one pouce below the occiput and two and a half fingers' breadth from the median line.
Stomach 36:	four fingers' breadth below the knee-cap, two fingers' breadth outside the tibial crest.
Urinary Bladder 18:	on the horizontal between the ninth and tenth dorsal vertebrae, one and a half pouces from the median line.

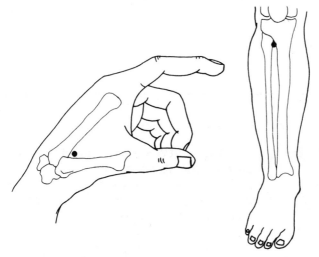

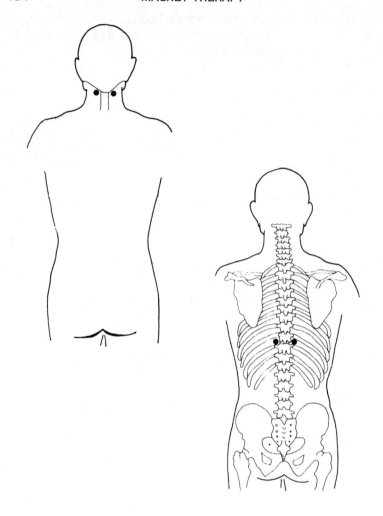

VERTIGO (MÉNIÈRE'S SYNDROME)

Jên-mai 12:   half-way between the navel and the
                  base of the sternum.

Stomach 36:   four fingers' breadth below the
                  kneecap, two fingers' breadth outside
                  the tibial crest. (See illustration on page
                  133).

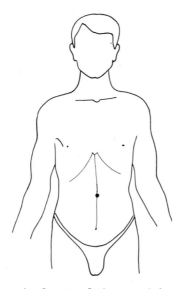

Small Intestine 19:	in front of the ear lobe and behind the temperomaxillary articulation.
Three Heaters 17:	in a hollow formed between the lobe and the mastoid bone when the mouth is opened.

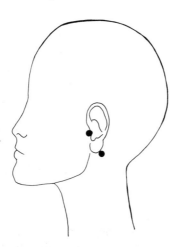

Gall Bladder 20:	one pouce below the occiput and two and a half fingers' breadth from the median line.

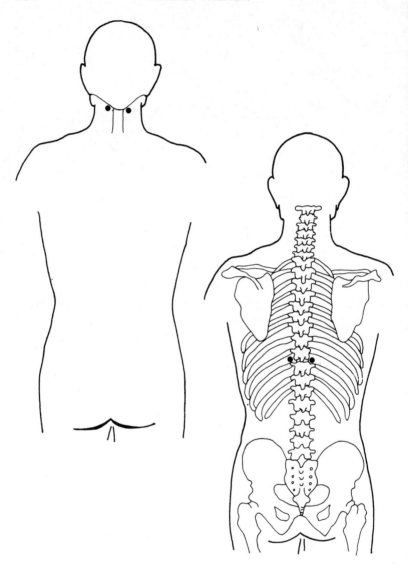

Urinary
Bladder 18: on the horizontal line passing between the ninth and tenth dorsal vertebrae, one and a half pouces from the median line.

6.

ADVICE TO PRACTITIONERS

Trained practitioners of acupuncture will be able to apply the magnetic pellets with a higher degree of refinement than described in the practical part of this book. They should take into account all the great energy laws employed in acupuncture: the circulation of energy, the balance of Yin and Yang, void and plenitude, protection of the organs and viscera, etc.

The magnetic pellets should prove very valuable in the treatment of children (under the age of seven they find the needles frightening) and of those who react badly to acupuncture – notably sufferers from spasmophilia and patients who have been given radiation (by cobalt or X-rays). In such cases, even the magnetic pellets must be used with caution and it is necessary to limit their number. When radiation has been given, treatment must be confined to the remote points, avoiding the irradiated zones. However, an acupuncture session with the magnetic pellets follows the same pattern as one where needles are employed. As we have seen earlier, the effect of a magnetic field on acupuncture points is not the same as that obtained by piqure; nor can we exactly duplicate tonification and dispersion by switching from one magnetic pole to the other.

In order to strike a proper balance between Yin and Yang, we can use the main Yin-Yang points, which may also be utilized according to the Issoujen's laws of imbrication of Yin and Yang.

It will always be helpful to act on the special meridians, especially on their centres of energy. The action of the magetic pellet is more to 'open' the points known as centres of energy than to tonify or disperse Yin or Yang.

The law of the five elements, and the Shen and K'o energy cycles, may also be used to great advantage with the magnetic pellets. By selecting the appropriate seasonal point of tonification or dispersion in the Shen energy cycle (and this will have an effect whatever the technique of stimulation chosen) we can lead the energy to or from the organ concerned in keeping with the cycle. The points of protection for given elements against other 'aggressive' elements in the K'o cycles can also be treated by magnetic pellets.

The well-known points for the treatment of disturbed energy in a main meridian, and the points of command in the Three Heaters, are equally available for the magnetic pellets (always excepting the Ting points at the tips of the fingers or toes, where naturally one refrains from placing them).

The treatment of mental disorders — in those who would not tolerate the needles — can also be simplified by using the magnetic pellets in accordance with the law of the five elements and of the visceral entities, or by utilizing specific points.

And so, the magnetic pellets can in certain cases be subsituted for the needles, in the same way as one can substitute manual or electrical stimulation or moxas, and obtain distinctive results from each method.

Magnetic pellets may also be used to prolong therapy if placed on the most important points treated at a session. For several days the magnetic field will continue the action initiated by the needle and will help the body to settle down into a new state of balance.

CONCLUSION

The application of magnetic pellets to the acupuncture points is an original procedure bridging the gap between methods thousands of years old such as acupuncture, or hundreds of years old such as magnet therapy, and methods springing from more recent interests such as natural medicine and our new understanding of magnetic phenomena and of the *modus operandi* of acupuncture. What is more, the application of a magnetic field has the virtues of simplicity, freedom from danger and low cost. Not only is the application of magnetic pellets a valuable aid to the therapist, whether acupuncturist of kinesitherapist; it offers the lay man or woman a suitable form of self-treatment for the minor ills of everyday life.

The fixed relationships studied in this book between points of imbalance in the internal organs (also reflected in mental states) and projection points on the surface of the body, come into play quite clearly during the application of magnetic pellets — an application not merely empirical but based on understanding. Therefore let us stress the intelligent nature of the treatment, since diagnosis and cure should go hand in hand even though they are too often separated in medicine, which may attempt to treat symptoms without comprehending the root of the malady or may comprehend causes without offering adequate treatment for their effects.

Obviously, we do not yet know everything about the mode of action of a polarized magnetic field placed on the surface of the body, nor everything about the complex variations in energy that can be induced through the stimulation of acupuncture points. Nevertheless, recent research into the relationship between the laws of acupuncture and chronobiology and into the possible link between changes in the earth's magnetic field and pathological conditions peculiar to our century, leads us to expect an ever-growing interest in these matters. Other research leans in the same direction, and the interest must surely be encouraged by the fact that the magnetic pellets are so easy to use and so beneficial.

BIBLIOGRAPHY

Durville, H., *Pour combattre les maladies par l'application de l'aimant* (Fighting disease by the application of magnets). (Nouvelle Edition Perthuis, 1971).

Davis, A.R. and Rawls, W.C., *Magnetism and its effects on the living system* (Exposition Press, New York, 1974).

Davis, A.R. and Rawls, W.C., *The Magnetic Effect* (Exposition Press, New York, 1974).

Sierra., and Bhattacharia., *Power in a magnet to heal* (Bhattacharia, India, 1976).

Yamada, A., *A Study on the Treatment effects of Magnetic Necklaces and their influence on living bodies*, (Shunichi Hirose, Internal Physiotherapy School, Medical Faculty, the University of Tokyo).

Barnothy., *Biological effects of magnetic fields* (University of New York, 1964).

INDEX